A SOURCEBOOK OF
HIV/AIDS PREVENTION
PROGRAMS
VOLUME 2

EDUCATION SECTOR–WIDE APPROACHES

Edited by
Michael Beasley
Alexandria Valerio
Donald A. P. Bundy

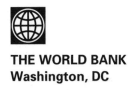

THE WORLD BANK
Washington, DC

ISBN: 978-0-8213-7440-5
eISBN: 978-0-8213-7441-2
DOI: 10.1596/978-0-8213-7440-5

Library of Congress Cataloging-in-Publication Data

A sourcebook of HIV/AIDS prevention programs. volume 2, Education sector-wide approaches / edited by Michael Beasley, Alexandria Valerio, Don Bundy.
   p. ; cm.
   Volume 1 has title: Education and HIV/AIDS.
   Includes bibliographical references.
   ISBN 978-0-8213-7440-5 (alk. paper) — ISBN 978-0-8213-7441-2 (electronic)
   1. AIDS (Disease)—Africa—Prevention. I. Beasley, Michael, 1968- II. Valerio, Alexandria, 1968- III. Bundy, Donald A. P. IV. Education and HIV/AIDS.
   [DNLM: 1. HIV Infections—prevention & control—Resource Guides. 2. Acquired Immunodeficiency Syndrome—prevention & control—Resource Guides. 3. Health Education—Resource Guides. WC 39 S724 2008]
   RA643.86.A35E385 2008
   616.97.9205096—dc22

2007047526

Cover design: Quantum Think, based on an earlier design by Rock Creek Publishing Group
Cover photograph: Amanda Koster Photography

A SOURCEBOOK OF
HIV/AIDS PREVENTION PROGRAMS

VOLUME 2

EDUCATION SECTOR–WIDE APPROACHES

Contents

Boxes

Figures

Tables

Preface

In recent years the education sector has played an increasingly important role in the prevention of HIV. Staying in school and getting a good education are now recognized as making an important contribution to helping young people, especially girls, avoid infection. Children of school age have the lowest prevalence of HIV, and even in the worst-affected countries the vast majority of schoolchildren remain uninfected. For these children there is a window of hope, a chance of a life free from HIV/AIDS if they acquire the knowledge, skills, and values to help protect themselves as they grow up. Providing young people with the "social vaccine" of education offers them a real chance of a productive life.

Not only is education important in preventing infection: preventing HIV is essential for education. By affecting education supply, demand, and quality, the HIV epidemic is limiting the capacity of countries to achieve Education for All (EFA) and the Millennium Development Goals (MDGs), and in the worst affected countries we are witnessing a reversal of hard-won educational gains.

This book was produced in response to demand from the readers of the first volume in this series, which largely reported on advocacy programs and on a relatively few, and rather small-scale interventions, often as pilots. The programs described in the new volume reflect the changing character of the education sector's response to HIV/AIDS. Since 2003, the focus has shifted to large-scale, effective implementation at the national level. Ministries of education across Africa and beyond are playing an increasingly active role in the national multisectoral response to HIV.

The previous volume was one of the most widely disseminated and popular titles among the hundreds of thousands of documents on HIV and education distributed through World Bank–supported projects. We hope that the present volume will prove to be an equally popular and effective source of information for those planning multisectoral responses to HIV, and will assist the development of even more programs that will help children grow up free of infection.

Elizabeth Laura Lule
Manager
AIDS Campaign Team
  for Africa
Africa Region
The World Bank

Debrework Zewdie
Director
Global HIV/AIDS
  Program
Human Development
  Network
The World Bank

Ruth Kagia
Director
Education Sector
Human Development
  Network
The World Bank

Acknowledgments

This document was prepared by Michael Beasley, Esther Miedema, Anthi Patrikios, and Lesley Drake of the Partnership for Child Development (Department of Infectious Disease Epidemiology, Imperial College, United Kingdom) under the technical leadership of Alexandria Valerio and Don Bundy of the education team at the World Bank. We appreciated the overall support of Yaw Ansu, Ruth Kagia, Debrework Zewdie, Dzingai Mutumbuka, Jee-Peng Tan, and Aidan Mulkeen (all the World Bank). Production of the Sourcebook was supported by Irish Aid.

We are grateful to Toyin Akpan (Consultant, Nigeria), Kiflay Andemichael (MoE, Eritrea), Helen Baños Smith (Consultant, United Kingdom), Cynthia Bosumtwi-Sam (MoESS, Ghana), Criana Connal (Consultant, United Kingdom), Pascaline Dupas (Abdul Latif Jameel Poverty Action Lab, United States), Hilda Eghan (MoESS, Ghana), Nike Esiet (AHI, Nigeria), Uwem Esiet (AHI, Nigeria), Clara Fayorsey (Consultant, Ghana), Silke Felton (UNICEF, Namibia), Alicia Fentiman (Consultant, United Kingdom), Willa Friedman (Abdul Latif Jameel Poverty Action Lab, United States), Mary Gichuru (CfBT, Kenya), Mussie Habte Ghebretinsae (MoE, Eritrea), Arisa Hernández (SEE, Dominican Republic), Sherif Yunus Hydara (DOSE, The Gambia), Silvia Jonas (Consultant, Israel), Albert Kpoor (Consultant, Ghana), Michael Kremer (Abdul Latif Jameel Poverty Action Lab, United States), Negusse Maekele (MoE, Eritrea), Amicoleh Mbaye (DOSE, The Gambia), Cristina Molina (SEE, Dominican Republic), Wairimu Muita (Consultant, Kenya), Rushnan Murtaza (UNICEF, Namibia), Obatunde Oladapo (Consultant, Nigeria), Hanni Oren (JAIP, Israel), Eccoua Oyinloye (MoEST, Nigeria), Mary Quaye (MoESS, Ghana), Inon Schenker (JAIP, Israel), Shamani-Jeffrey Shikwambi (Consultant, Namibia), Lucy Steinitz (MoE, Namibia), Vincent Tay (Consultant, Ghana), William Vargas (Consultant, Dominican Republic), and Janet Wildish (CfBT, Kenya) for the collection of data and the support of activities in participating countries.

We appreciated the contributions of Florian Fichtl, Michael Mills, Eunice Yaa Brimfah Dapaah, Joe Valadez, and Christopher Walker (all from the World Bank), who facilitated the collection of data and contributed to the analysis.

Many other people contributed to discussions of the issues considered here and to the reviewing process: David Clarke (independent consultant), Amaya Gillespie (UNSG's Study on Violence Against Children), Anna-Maria Hofmans (UNICEF), Matthew Jukes (Harvard University), Michael

Kelly (University of Zambia), Doug Kirby (ETR Associates), Seung-hee Lee (Save the Children USA), Stella Manda (World Bank), Sergio Meresman (CEDAPS), Christine Panchaud (IBE), and Andy Tembon (World Bank). The manuscript benefited from peer reviewer comments from Janet Leno and Albertus Voetberg of the World Bank.

We thank Barbara Karni for copyediting the Sourcebook, and Aziz Gökdemir, Paola Scalabrin, and Denise Bergeron (all at the World Bank's Office of the Publisher) for overseeing book production from start to finish.

Availability of the Sourcebook

The *Sourcebook* is available on the Internet, at http://www.schoolsand health.org and http://www.unesco.org/education/ibe/ichae.

French and Portuguese versions are planned for distribution on CD.

For further information or to order printed copies or CDs, contact the World Bank Education Advisory Service, at http://www.worldbank.org/ education.

You may also e-mail the Education Advisory Service at eservice@world bank.org or write to:

Education Advisory Service
The World Bank
1818 H Street, NW
Washington, DC 20433
USA

Abbreviations

ABC	Abstinence, Being faithful, and Condom use
ACU	AIDS Control Unit
AHI	Action Health Incorporated
AIDS	acquired immunodeficiency syndrome
ARFH	Association for Reproductive and Family Health
CBO	community-based organization
CDC	Centers for Disease Control and Prevention
CfBT	Centre for British Teachers
CIDA	Canadian International Development Agency
COPRESIDA	Presidential Council on HIV/AIDS
CSO	civil society organization
DANIDA	Danish International Development Agency
DFID	Department for International Development
DoSE	Department of State for Education
ECOWAS	Economic Community of West African States
EFA	Education for All
ELPE	Expanded Life Planning Education
FBO	faith-based organization
FLHE	Family Life HIV/AIDS Education
GAC	Ghana AIDS Commission
GAMET	Global Monitoring and Evaluation Team
GDP	Gross Domestic Product
GES	Ghana Education Service
HAART	Highly Active Antiretroviral Therapy
HAMSET	HIV/AIDS, Malaria, STDs, and Tuberculosis Project Management Unit
HAMU	HIV/AIDS Management Unit
HIV	human immunodeficiency virus
ICS	International Child Support
IDF	Israeli Defense Forces
JAIP	Jerusalem AIDS Project
JICA	Japan International Cooperation Agency
KAP	Knowledge, Attitude, and Practice
KAPB	Knowledge, Attitudes, Practices, and Beliefs
KIE	Kenya Institute of Education
LPE	life-planning education
LQAS	Lot Quality Assurance Sampling
LSMoE	Lagos State Ministry of Education
MBESC	Ministry of Basic Education, Sport and Culture
MDGs	Millennium Development Goals
M&E	monitoring and evaluation
MIT	Massachusetts Institute of Technology
MoESS	Ministry of Education, Science, and Sports
MoEST	Ministry of Education, Science, and Technology
NACC	National AIDS Control Council

NAS	National AIDS Secretariat
NERDC	Nigerian Education Research and Development Council
NGO	nongovernmental organization
NIED	National Institute for Educational Development
NSGA	Nova Scotia–Gambia Association
ODA	Overseas Development Agency (U.K.)
PAHO	Pan American Health Organization
PCD	Partnership for Child Development
PEAS	Programa de Educación Afectivo Sexual
POP/FLE	Population and Family Life Education
PP TESCOM	Post Primary Teaching Service Commission (renamed the Teachers Establishment and Pensions Office [TEPO])
PRISM	Primary School Management program
PROCETS	Programa de Control de Enfermedades de Transmisión Sexual y SIDA
PSABH	Primary School Action for Better Health
PTA	parent-teacher association
RHS&A	Robert H. Schaffer & Associates
RRI	Rapid Results Initiative
SEE	State Secretariat of Education
SHAPE	Strengthening HIV/AIDS Partnership in Education
SHEP	School Health Education Program
SMC	school management committee
SQAD	Standard and Quality Assurance Directorate
STDs	sexually transmitted diseases
STI	sexually transmitted infection
TASO	The AIDS Support Organization
TESCOM	Teaching Service Commission
UNAIDS	Joint United Nations Programme on HIV/AIDS
UNDP	United Nations Development Programme
UNFPA	United Nations Family Planning Association
UNICEF	United Nations Children's Fund
USAID	United States Agency for International Development
WHO	World Health Organization
WoH	Window of Hope

Introduction

In response to the education sector's demand for information, in 2004, the World Bank produced a *Sourcebook of HIV/AIDS Prevention Programs*. That volume documented education-based prevention programs targeting children and youth in seven countries in Sub-Saharan Africa. Most of the programs included were small and occurred in nonformal settings. Others concentrated on the production and dissemination of information and educational, and communication materials. Few were led by ministries of education, and none was part of the formal curriculum. The programs documented were typical of the education sector response to HIV/AIDS at the time.

Feedback received during the review and use of the first sourcebook suggested that because school systems reach large numbers of young people and have the infrastructure to deliver large-scale, cost-effective education, it would be useful to document school-based programs led by ministries of education. A second phase of work was proposed that focused on identifying and documenting school-based approaches that are appropriate in cost and scope for implementation by the public sector.

This volume describes 10 school-based HIV prevention programs (table 1). Unlike the first volume, it includes programs from non-African countries that have relevance to Africa. All of the programs are school based and involve teachers; target school-age children; are considered successful, well implemented, and innovative; and have the potential to be replicated and scaled up.

In order to develop the Sourcebook, the Partnership for Child Development (PCD)—the organization that acted as the secretariat charged with production of the Sourcebook—sent requests for information on programs to more than 30 experts in education sector–based HIV prevention.[1] Programs that met the inclusion criteria were included on a shortlist, which the international experts reviewed. The shortlist included as wide a variety of different program approaches as possible, including programs based on curriculum-based teaching, extracurricular activities, and peer education.

The Sourcebook's findings are based on the responses to three sets of questionnaires administered to program managers and implementers, as well as a questionnaire administered to student participants. Responses to the program description questionnaire described the rationale, aims and objectives, target audience, components, and main approaches of each program. Responses to the implementation questionnaire described the program's process, from the initial needs assessment through the development of materials and training to the practical details of implementation. They

Table 1: Program Descriptions

COUNTRY	PROGRAM	PROGRAM DESCRIPTION
Dominican Republic	Programa de Educación Afectivo Sexual (PEAS)	Sex education with strong component on sexually transmitted infections, including HIV, integrated into curriculum in all secondary-school grades
Eritrea	Rapid Results Initiative© (RRI)	Rapid implementation of school-based extracurricular HIV prevention activities
Gambia, The	Integrated Sector-Wide HIV/AIDS Preventive Education	Country-level education sector response to HIV/AIDS coordinated by the Department of State for Education and implemented by a range of partners
Ghana	School Health Education Program (SHEP)	Government-coordinated school-based HIV/AIDS education implemented by range of governmental and nongovernmental stakeholders
Israel	Jerusalem AIDS Project (JAIP)	Volunteer-provided HIV/AIDS extracurricular education for primary- and secondary-school students
Kenya	Primary School Action for Better Health (PSABH)	Teacher-led HIV/AIDS and behavior change education for students aged 12–16
Kenya	Primary School AIDS Prevention	Randomized assessment of impact of different approaches aimed at reducing risky behavior among adolescents
Namibia	Window of Hope (WoH)	Extracurricular HIV/AIDS and life-skills education tailored to needs of different age groups
Nigeria	Expanded Life Planning Education (ELPE)	Curricular and extracurricular HIV/AIDS and life-skills education
Nigeria	National Family Life HIV/AIDS Education (FLHE)	HIV/AIDS and life-skills teaching integrated into two main carrier subjects in regular curriculum for junior-secondary school students

Source: Authors.

also provided information on the finances of each program, which in some cases are used to estimate unit costs. Responses to a third questionnaire provided insights on challenges and lessons learned and the extent to which the program complied with a set of characteristics of effective programs drawn from an initial analysis of 83 evaluations of sex and HIV education programs in developing and developed countries, later published as Kirby, Laris, and Rolleri (2005).

The Sourcebook is organized as follows. Each program is described in its own chapter, which begins with "at-a-glance" information and ends with an assessment of program performance on a set of impact benchmarks and contact information. The four main sections of each chapter—program description, implementation, research and evaluation, and lessons learned—provide readers with a thorough sense of each intervention and its applicability to other settings.

Discussion of the curricular approach in each chapter examines how HIV/AIDS education is integrated into the school curriculum. This integration usually takes one (or a combination) of five forms:[2]

- *Stand-alone subject.* The topic is clearly labeled and included in the school curriculum. It addresses all issues relevant to HIV prevention and mitigation.

- *Integrated in one main carrier subject.* Teaching and learning of most of the relevant material is addressed within one main carrier subject, such as social science, family education, or biology.

- *Cross-curricular subject.* The topic is integrated in a limited number of subjects (in no more than one-third of all subjects in the curriculum). HIV/AIDS teaching and learning within these few subjects is clearly divided across carrier subjects.

- *Infused throughout the curriculum.* The topic is integrated into a wide range of subjects.

- *Extracurricular or co-curricular topic.* Schools sponsor extracurricular activities, which may be taught during the regular school day or after school. Course credit is rarely given for these activities. Some programs also offer co-curricular activities (activities that complement or reinforce the regular curriculum), for which students can receive credit.

Notes

1. Created in 1992, the Partnership for Child Development is committed to improving the education, health, and nutrition of school-age children and youth in low-income countries. It is based within the Department of Infectious Disease Epidemiology in the Faculty of Medicine at London's Imperial College. The organization helps countries and international agencies turn the findings of evidence-based research into national interventions that benefit children around the world.

2. Definitions of curricular approaches are based on those described in IBE-UNESCO (2005). See also IBE-UNESCO (2006). The terms used to describe the different approaches vary across countries. For consistency the definitions shown here are used throughout.

References

IBE-UNESCO. 2005. *The Quality Imperative: Assessment of Curricular Response in 35 Countries for the EFA Monitoring Report 2005.* Geneva: IBE-UNESCO. Available at http://unesdoc.unesco.org/ulis/cgi-bin/ulis.pl?by=2&ca=ibe&look=ibe&req=2&text=primaires.

———. 2006. *Manual for Integrating HIV and AIDS Education in School Curricula.* Geneva: IBE-UNESCO. Available at http://www.ibe.unesco.org/AIDS/Manual/Manual_home.htm.

Kirby, D., B. A. Laris, and L. Rolleri. 2005. "Impact of Sex and HIV Education Programs on Sexual Behaviors of Youth in Developing and Developed Countries." FHI Working Paper Series No. 2, Family Health International, Triangle Park, N.C.

PEAS at a Glance

Description: Program integrates HIV/AIDS education into the secondary-school curriculum to improve knowledge and change values, attitudes, and behavior of teachers and students. Program covers prevention and transmission of sexually transmitted infections (STIs), including HIV, as well as promotion of human rights and gender equality, with a view to reinforcing students' capacity to make conscious and responsible decisions.

Number of schools participating: 825 secondary schools, at which 10,098 teachers implement the program.

Coverage: Countrywide, covering 73 percent of all secondary-school students.

Target groups: Program currently targets secondary-school students. Intention is eventually to reach all students in the national education system.

Components: The program consists of six main components: education on STIs, including HIV; advocacy and building of intersectoral partnerships; development of materials; teacher training and support; community outreach; and research and development.

Establishment and duration: Begun in 2001, ongoing.

Management: Department of Counseling and Psychology of State Secretariat of Education (SEE) and the Presidential Council on HIV/AIDS (COPRESIDA).

Key partners: Program is supported by a multidisciplinary and multisectoral team that includes staff from the education, health, labor, youth affairs, science and technology, women's affairs, and tourism ministries. Government authorities also work in close partnership with a range of bilateral and multilateral organizations, international and national NGOs, and religious authorities.

Costs: Not provided.

Key evaluation results: Knowledge about HIV/AIDS was found to increase with grade. Evaluation demonstrated both program successes (e.g., that most students abstain from sex or use condoms) and challenges (e.g., views about HIV/AIDS where common myths endure).

Programa de Educación Afectivo Sexual (PEAS), the Dominican Republic

HIV/AIDS has taken a terrible toll in the Dominican Republic (box 1.1), but the country has emerged as a regional "success story" in recent years. National prevention and control strategies have resulted in measurable reductions in the number of sexual partners and increased condom use, reducing the risk of HIV infection.

To respond to the epidemic, the government of the Dominican Republic created a high-level political institution, the Presidential Council on HIV/AIDS (COPRESIDA), which reports directly to the president and coordinates the fight against the epidemic. COPRESIDA approaches the epidemic from multiple perspectives—economic, social, and cultural—involving various sectors and actors through partnerships with government, the private sector, and civil society organizations (CSOs), including people living with HIV/AIDS.

As the epidemic has evolved, COPRESIDA has strengthened and expanded successful strategies, including increasing voluntary counseling and testing, controlling sexually transmitted infections (STIs), reducing mother-to-child transmission, and providing care and treatment according to established guidelines for people with HIV who require it. These strategies promote cost-effective interventions, targeting the most vulnerable groups. As part of this multisectoral approach, the Programa de Educación Afectivo Sexual (Sex Education Program) was launched in 2001 in Santa Domingo, which has the highest prevalence of HIV/AIDS and the largest number of teen pregnancies in the country.

William Vargas, consultant, conducted the interviews and collected the data for this chapter. Arisa Hernández and Cristina Molina, of the PEAS Program, provided support, encouragement, and assistance. Criana Connal, consultant, assisted in drafting the text of this chapter.

Box 1.1: Facts and Figures on HIV/AIDS in the Dominican Republic

---

- About 20,000 people died from AIDS-related illnesses between 1994 and 2004.
- An estimated 120,000 people were living with HIV/AIDS in 2004, nine times the total number of reported cases.
- Heterosexual intercourse accounts for 81 percent of HIV cases among 15- to 44-year-olds. The fact that the Dominican Republic is a major tourist destination may partly account for the high rate of infection.
- Prevalence is highest (5 percent of adults) among low-income groups, including many Haitian immigrants living in rural communities and working on sugar cane plantations. Prevalence among female commercial sex workers is about 8 percent, reaching 12 percent in some cities.
- AIDS is the leading cause of death among women of reproductive age. Underlying problems include high rates of sexually transmitted infections (STIs), high birth rates among adolescent girls and young women, and active migration between cities and the countryside as well as from Haiti.
- Tuberculosis is the largest opportunistic infection for people living with AIDS. The Pan American Health Organization (PAHO) estimates that more than 100 per 100,000 people are infected with tuberculosis. These figures are orders of magnitude higher than in nearby countries, such as Barbados (2.6 per 100,000) and Jamaica (4.9 per 100,000). The 5,320 reported cases in the Dominican Republic in 2004 were among the highest in the Latin America and Caribbean region.

Source: World Bank/COPRESIDA 2004a.

Description

The Programa de Educación Afectivo Sexual (PEAS) is an innovative response to HIV/AIDS by two state organs, the State Secretariat of Education (SEE) and COPRESIDA. Through integration into the school curriculum, the program aims to reinforce knowledge and change values, attitudes, and behavior of teachers and students at all levels of the system, starting with secondary schools. The program covers prevention and transmission of STIs, including HIV, as well as the promotion of human rights and gender equality, with a view to reinforcing students' capacity to make conscious and responsible decisions.

Rationale and History

PEAS staff estimated that in 2005 about half of all adolescents and youth in the Dominican Republic—some 783,000 people—had not received sex education. The need for such education was evident: in 1996 almost a quarter of adolescent girls were pregnant or had given birth. Unplanned pregnancies at a very early age heighten maternal and child health risks and limit the psychosocial development of young men and women.

The prevalence of STIs is increasing in the Dominican Republic. The mass media and chauvinist cultural patterns promote a one-dimensional concept of sexuality (that is, the expression of sexual passion). At the same time, a lack of timely information about sexuality, sexual and reproductive health, and STIs and the lack of communication within the family place young people in a vulnerable position when confronted with these challenges.

The country's National Strategic Plan for 2000–04 declared sex education in schools a high priority. The plan, developed in light of a statement made by the government of the Dominican Republic during the June 2001 United Nations General Assembly Special Session on HIV/AIDS, committed the government to the following actions over a five-year period:

- Develop a sex education program that targets adolescents.

- Create a strategic alliance with the pharmaceutical industry to produce generic antiretroviral medications at an affordable price.

- Implement a national policy to promote and distribute condoms to vulnerable populations.

- Expand mother-to-child transmission prevention efforts throughout the public health system (USAID 2002).

This commitment is supported by Law 5593, promulgated in 1995, which specifies the rights of people infected with HIV and the duties of employers, doctors, and others who interact with them. Nongovernmental organizations (NGOs) are now trying to monitor the law's enforcement.

In August 2001 SEE, the department in charge of planning for and administering the national educational system, launched PEAS (figure 1.1). The program's design and development took place within the context of the Dominican Republic's HIV/AIDS Prevention and Control Project (Programa de Control de Enfermedades de Transmisión Sexual y SIDA [PROCETS]), launched in February 2002 (box 1.2). It resides within the Public Health State Office of the Secretary of Social Aid.

Figure 1.1: Timeline of PEAS Development

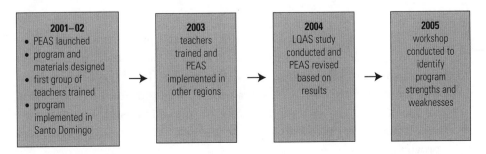

Source: Authors.

Box 1.2: The Dominican Republic's HIV/AIDS Prevention and Control Project

The $30 million HIV/AIDS Prevention and Control Project was launched in the Dominican Republic in 2002, under the World Bank–financed $155 million multicountry HIV/AIDS Prevention and Control Program for the Caribbean Region. Implementation partners include the Global Fund for HIV/AIDS, Tuberculosis, and Malaria; the U.S. Agency for International Development; the Clinton Foundation; the Pan American Health Organization/World Health Organization; the United Nations Development Programme (UNDP); and Partners for Health.
  The project has three main components:

1. *Activities to prevent HIV transmission.* Activities include information, education, and communication activities and social marketing of condoms, particularly among vulnerable groups. A multisectoral approach is ensured by participation agreements with 13 government ministries, including the ministries of education, labor, youth affairs, science and technology, women's affairs, and tourism; 4 military and police agencies; 4 civil society organizations (CSOs); 3 private sector groups; and 2 religious groups. The mother-to-child transmission program, initiated in 1999, covers all public hospitals providing maternity services and 83 percent of health centers and municipal facilities. In 2004 the program reached about 157,000 (78 percent) of the estimated 200,000 pregnant women in the country. The program also promotes the social marketing of condoms, the strengthening of activities that prevent and control tuberculosis, and a pilot HIV prevention and control project in tourist areas. Baseline surveys of special population groups, including commercial sex workers, men who have sex with men, Haitian immigrants living in *bateyes* (areas around sugar cane plantations), and prisoners have provided key information for designing interventions to target these groups.

2. *Diagnosis, basic care, and support of people affected by HIV/AIDS.* This component seeks to reduce disability and death, decrease transmission of HIV/AIDS, and support children orphaned by AIDS. It includes the Highly Active Antiretroviral Therapy (HAART) Treatment Program, established through the Comprehensive Care Central Unit of the Ministry of Health. This program aims to cover 20,000 people between 2005 and 2008.

3. *Support for stronger surveillance systems, project coordination, monitoring and evaluation, and research.* The project has conducted behavioral and biological surveys of high-risk groups, geographic mapping of vulnerable groups in Puerto Plata, and sentinel seroprevalence surveys. Criteria, indicators, and methods for monitoring and evaluating impact have been streamlined within a coherent framework.

Source: World Bank/COPRESIDA 2004.

On January 24, 2002, COPRESIDA signed a participation agreement with SEE, to develop the PEAS for secondary-school students to counter the expansion of HIV among 15- to 19-year-olds. The HIV/AIDS prevention unit was created in SEE, and a process of sensitization was developed to reach officials at various levels of the administrative hierarchy, supplemented by the training of officials at the central, regional, and provincial levels.

Objectives

The PEAS objectives include the following:

- Promote healthy sexual behaviors and facilitate informed decision making by children and youth.

- Increase young people's knowledge about sexual and reproductive health.

- Develop positive attitudes concerning self-esteem, self-awareness, confidence, and respect and values for self and others.

- Combat the stigma surrounding HIV/AIDS.

- Decrease the number of sexual partners.

- Delay the age of sexual initiation.

- Prevent HIV/AIDS, other STIs, and teenage pregnancies.

- Promote public health policy.

Strategies

The program's main strategy is to teach sex education, with a strong STI and HIV/AIDS component, to all students in all four years of secondary school. The program promotes sexual abstinence, safe sex, and condom use; discourages teenage pregnancies; and encourages communication between young adults and their parents.

On the basis of the results of a survey carried out in 2004 (described below), the PEAS program developed a strategic plan. The plan outlines the aims and implementation strategies of the program and provides teacher guidelines. On the basis of the survey, a number of recommendations were made for strengthening the program:

- Set up a peer education component aimed at providing peer support and counseling.

- Involve parents and caregivers in the program.

- Integrate income-generating activities.

- Create supportive environments.

- Support community action for health change, community outreach, and mobilization.

- Promote and conserve positive cultural and traditional arts and modes of communication.

- Increase the capacity of NGO staff to deal with HIV/AIDS and sexual health issues in their own programs.

To implement these strategies, PEAS uses audio-visual presentations, focus group discussions, role-play, brainstorming sessions, dramatization, parent-teacher meetings, talks and lectures, visits and interactions with people living with HIV/AIDS, and games.

Target Groups

Public secondary-school students are currently the main target group. As of 2004, 73 percent of all students enrolled in secondary school in the Dominican Republic had participated in PEAS. The program intends to expand to reach all students in the national education system, beginning with preschool and extending to the postsecondary level.

Philosophy and Components

PEAS is based on the belief that the best ways to prevent HIV in children and youth are to:

• understand the knowledge, attitudes, and sexual practices of students;

• involve students, parents, and teachers in designing a prevention program;

• integrate the program into the curriculum of all schools that are part of the national education system;

• teach children about the dangers of having sex at an early age

• break the myth about AIDS not being real.

The program consists of six main components, which build on and complement one another:

• STI and HIV/AIDS education

• Advocacy and building of intersectoral partnerships

• Development of materials

• Teacher training and support

• Community outreach

• Research and development

Program messages are integrated into the national curriculum and delivered during school hours. The program is managed by each school's counseling and psychology unit. The program employs a holistic approach (see figure 1.2) and aims to support students in developing skills and values,

Figure 1.2: Basic Aspects of the PEAS Program

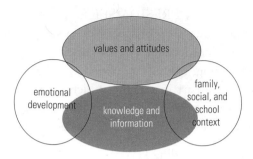

values and attitudes

emotional development

knowledge and information

family, social, and school context

Source: Authors.

such as the value of self-care, respect for life and responsibility, and the value of sexual abstinence. Students are also provided with information on contraception, including the use of condoms as a means to prevent STIs and pregnancy. School counselors and psychologists, many of whom received university-level training in HIV/AIDS and sex education, support teachers delivering the program.

Implementation

To raise awareness about the aims and strategies of the program and the needs to which it responds, PEAS carried out a process of awareness-raising among officials at various levels in the administrative hierarchy. It supplemented these activities by training officials at the central, regional, and provincial levels.

Through a series of meetings between SEE and COPRESIDA, the structure and content of PEAS were finalized. The program was then offered to all secondary schools as part of the regular curriculum. Teachers and principals are responsible for implementing the PEAS education component and ensuring that it reaches students and their families. The principal has ultimate responsibility for ensuring that the PEAS curriculum is implemented.

The Ministry of Education is responsible for implementing PEAS. Funding decisions are made by COPRESIDA, however, which manages the funds allocated by the World Bank for HIV/AIDS–related policies. This structure can be challenging, because the Ministry of Education does not have easy access to funds and cannot always respond adequately to new needs.

Training

Between 2001 and 2005, COPRESIDA/SEE formed a multidisciplinary team of training facilitators, made up of specialists in sex education, psychology, counseling, and medicine. Secondary-school teachers received training in the delivery of PEAS during a three-day period. Teachers from all disciplines were welcomed to take part in training, which used a variety of methods, including lectures, case analyses, group discussions, experience-sharing, and audio-visual presentations. Topics covered included the following:

- Prevention of STIs, including HIV

- Teenage pregnancy

- Domestic violence

- Drugs and delinquency

- Sexuality, values, and taboos

- Stigma and discrimination

- Solidarity with people living with HIV/AIDS.

In 2004 PEAS began training other school professionals (including school counselors and psychologists) as well as peer educators (table 1.1). It also began to offer refresher training, which gave previously trained teachers the opportunity to exchange ideas and experiences, strengthen their knowledge of HIV/AIDS–related sex education, and benefit from exposure to new concepts and information.

Teaching

Comprehensive sexuality and HIV/AIDS education is taught as a part of lessons in a variety of courses, including environmental and applied science,

Table 1.1: Number of People Who Received PEAS Training, 2001–05

ITEM	NUMBER TRAINED
Secondary-school teachers	10,098
Program trainers at the national level	35
Program trainers at the regional and district levels	118
Counselors and psychologists	1,800
Sexologists and physicians	40
School policy makers	200
Peer educators	1,280
Parents and family members	412
Total	13,983

Source: SEE 2006; PEAS Training 2001/2005.

biology, social studies, and health education, as well as through school counseling. In social sciences, natural sciences, and "comprehensive humanistic and religious education," the program emphasizes the foundations of sexuality and HIV/AIDS education. In counseling and parts of the curriculum that touch on psychology, ethics, and health education, sexuality is addressed from a cross-disciplinary perspective. This approach guarantees that education on sexuality is given from a biological, psychological, sociocultural, and spiritual point of view. The program pays a great deal of attention to the role of values in sexual education, in line with the goals and principles of education in the Dominican Republic (Education Law 66 1997).

Teaching focuses on four main areas: knowledge and information, attitudes and moral values, emotional development, and social (including family, school, and community) development. Specific topics addressed include the following:

- Sexual and reproductive health

- Prevention of STIs, including HIV

- Responsible sexual behavior (responsibility toward oneself and others)

- Sexual behavior from an emotional perspective

- Self-efficacy and self-esteem

- Responses to peer pressure

- Interpersonal communication skills, including parent-child communication

- Problem-solving skills

- Negotiating skills and the right to say no to sex (with emphasis on the rights of girls)

- Gender equality

- Attitudes toward sexual violence

- Protective skills

- The right to privacy, confidentiality, and informed consent

- Child rights, child abuse, and respect for others' rights

- Law 136-03 and the Code of Protection.

Teaching combines science-based information as well as discussion of the human side of HIV/AIDS, allowing students to connect the issue to real life. Students are informed not only about symptoms and the ways in which HIV/AIDS and other STIs are transmitted and prevented but also about taboos, myths, stigma, and discrimination. Students are also equipped with various life skills needed to cope in an environment in which the threat and prevalence of HIV/AIDS is high.

Age-appropriate PEAS instruction is given once a week, for 30–50 minutes, throughout the school year. Teachers are encouraged to integrate PEAS issues into their respective disciplines, depending on their teaching load and instruction time available.

The program has developed instructional media and pedagogical resources that can facilitate the teaching of cross-disciplinary contents. The main methods used by teachers are lectures, group discussions, and drama. Activities are designed to be participatory.

Sex education was long taboo in the Dominican Republic. After implementing the program, however, most teachers are not embarrassed to teach it. According to program officials, teaching the PEAS curriculum helps them review and improve their own attitudes and values about sexuality and HIV prevention.

Materials

All teachers are provided with a set of grade-appropriate materials. Materials include two main manuals, developed in 2001 and 2002 by a multidisciplinary team of health and education specialists from SEE and COPRESIDA, including experts from national universities. Teenagers were consulted during the development of the materials. The first manual, *Aprender a vivir* (*Learn How to Live*), consists of seven components, covering themes such as youth, sexuality, solidarity, and HIV/AIDS. The second manual, *Hablemos sobre sexualidad* (*Talking about Sexuality*), focuses on values, violence, self-esteem, and gender. These materials are used during both teacher training and classroom teaching. They also provide a variety of teaching and learning activities for NGOs and families. Supplementary resources—obtained from a variety of sources, including the Ministry of Health and national NGOs—are used by teachers both within and outside the formal school system to inform and support teaching.

Partnerships

Working under the aegis of COPRESIDA, PEAS is automatically part of a multidisciplinary and multisectoral team that includes staff from the education, health, labor, youth affairs, science and technology, women's affairs, and tourism ministries. In addition, government authorities work in close partnership with a range of bilateral and multilateral organizations and international and national NGOs.

Parents are involved in the program, and both teachers and students have identified their active participation as particularly important. Parental involvement varies across schools, however. In some communities parents take part in teacher-parent meetings and participate in training workshops. In others parents are not involved at all, because the program has targeted only students.

The active support of religious authorities has also been important. Some religious schools have solicited training from PEAS, which has been adapted for their use. Other religious schools, however, have taboos against teaching sex education and do not offer the program.

Student Evaluation

Evaluation of student progress is not done in a formal or systematic manner. Teachers informally assess student knowledge, attitudes, and skills by observing what students say and how they act during group discussions and other activities.

Teachers meet with the principal once a year to report on program progress. Central-level staff also hold meetings to evaluate the program. Technical personnel make use of the results of these sessions to improve the program.

Evaluation results (see below) have been used to strengthen program implementation strategies, to enhance the various themes, and to integrate new components. They have led to new activities, including a peer education program intended for teenagers and a training program for young leaders and the development of a series of teaching material and pedagogical methodologies intended for a variety of users.

Survey Results

In 2004 SEE and COPRESIDA sought technical assistance from the Global Monitoring and Evaluation Team (GAMET) of the World Bank to develop and administer a survey on knowledge of, attitudes toward, and practices related to STIs, HIV/AIDS, and sex education among students and secondary-school teachers and to evaluate the program. The survey was conducted in two regional education districts of Santo Domingo (regions 10 and 15).[1]

The Lot Quality Assurance Sampling (LQAS) method was used, with education districts representing supervision areas.[2] Twenty-seven members of the national technical team of SEE and COPRESIDA were trained in the LQAS methodology.[3]

The survey population consisted of public school students in grades 9–12 and teachers who were responsible for PEAS training in regions 10 and 15 of Santo Domingo. Random samples of students and teachers were selected from the school's student and teacher lists.[4] Indicators were developed based on the objectives for each grade (table 1.2).

In the six-month period studied, 52–64 percent of students in region 15 and 42–65 percent of students in region 10 received instruction on STIs, HIV/AIDS, and sex education at school. The distribution of educational materials was poor in the two regions, because the materials had not yet been edited; the few educational materials that were distributed had been photocopied. Despite having participated in some PEAS activities, students showed inadequate knowledge of the topics covered. Students had heard of STIs, for example, but many were confused about symptoms, transmission, treatment, and prevention.

Students demonstrated some knowledge regarding transmission of HIV/AIDS, although very few knew that HIV/AIDS can be transmitted from mother to child during birth or breastfeeding, and a large majority believe that the disease can be contracted by sharing a toilet with someone who is infected (table 1.3). Correct knowledge tended to increase with grade.

Table 1.2: PEAS Survey Indicators

KNOWLEDGE OF HIV PREVENTION	PRACTICES OF HIV PREVENTION
• Stated two or more ways of avoiding HIV • Stated at least one place where condoms could be obtained • Had heard about the HIV test • Cited at least one place where HIV tests could be performed	• Had sexual intercourse • Had sexual intercourse with more than one sexual partner during the previous 12 months • Used a condom during sexual intercourse • Used (or had partner use) a condom during first sexual intercourse • Used (or had partner use) a condom during most recent sexual intercourse • Had an HIV test • Would inform their partner if they had an HIV test

Source: World Bank/COPRESIDA 2004b.

Both boys and girls demonstrated knowledge of HIV prevention, and 5–18 percent of students indicated they had been tested for HIV. In all grades sexually active students tended to have only one partner. Most students abstain from sex or protect themselves by using a condom. Condom use increased by grade.

The survey revealed a prevalence of discriminatory attitudes and a lack of solidarity toward people living with HIV/AIDS. Large percentages of students would not permit a family member with HIV/AIDS to be taken care of in their home, and many believe that a person with HIV/AIDS should not continue to attend school.

Students recognized the responsibility of school and family in sex education and understood the dangers of teenage pregnancy. Many students considered pregnancy and the associated economic burden to be the responsibility of their family rather than themselves. Students were unable to use "correct" terms to identify male and female genitals, using popular terms instead.

The survey also provided several interesting findings on teachers:

- In the schools surveyed, only 25–62 percent of teachers had started implementing the program.

MYTHS AND PREJUDICES RELATED TO HIV/AIDS	TRAINING RECEIVED
• Would allow a family member with HIV/AIDS to be taken care of in their home • Would live with a family member with HIV/AIDS • Believe that a student with HIV/AIDS should remain in school • Do not believe that HIV/AIDS affects only prostitutes and homosexuals • Believe that people living with HIV/AIDS should not be isolated • Believe that HIV/AIDS is not a myth • Believe that a healthy-looking person can be infected with HIV • Believe that HIV is not transmitted by touching someone who is infected • Believe that HIV is not transmitted by mosquito bites • Believe that HIV is not transmitted by sharing a toilet with someone who is infected • Believe that HIV is not transmitted by sharing kitchen utensils with someone who is infected	• Attended talk at school about STIs/HIV/AIDS during previous six months • Received educational material at school about STIs/HIV/AIDS during previous six months • Participated in sociodrama or other type of educational activity at school about STIs/HIV/AIDS during previous six months at school.

Table 1.3: Student Knowledge of HIV/AIDS and Attitudes toward People Living with HIV/AIDS
(percent of all students)

| | FEMALE STUDENTS | | | | MALE STUDENTS | | | |
| | GRADE | | | | GRADE | | | |
INDICATOR	9	10	11	12	9	10	11	12
Knowledge of HIV/AIDS								
Believe that HIV/AIDS is not a myth	96	99	98	97	91	94	98	95
Believe that a healthy-looking person cannot be infected with HIV	77	86	94	92	91	80	91	95
Believe that HIV cannot be transmitted by mosquito bites	60	45	51	44	43	51	53	52
Believe that HIV cannot be transmitted by sharing kitchen utensils with an infected person	67	47	61	59	40	47	36	56
Believe that HIV cannot be transmitted by sharing a toilet with an infected person	29	28	39	36	36	33	25	40
Believe that HIV is not transmitted by touching an infected person	91	94	97	91	80	85	89	93
Attitudes toward people living with HIV/AIDS								
Would permit a family member with HIV/AIDS to be taken care of in their home	51	51	65	68	43	61	59	58
Would live with a family member having HIV/AIDS	55	52	70	75	46	55	64	65
Believe that a student with HIV/AIDS should remain in school	62	55	55	69	39	63	65	60
Believe that HIV/AIDS is not a disease that affects only prostitutes and homosexuals	86	86	91	97	75	85	85	95
Believe that people living with HIV/AIDS should not be isolated	83	85	89	89	68	72	84	85

Source: World Bank/COPRESIDA 2004b.

- Teachers' overall knowledge about sex education was satisfactory. However, many teachers did not recognize the economic burden borne by the family as a result of teenage pregnancy or the impact of teenage pregnancy on academic performance.

- Teachers recognized the responsibility of both school and family in delivering sex education; they considered themselves responsible actors of PEAS.

- Teachers showed adequate knowledge regarding prevention of HIV/AIDS and other STIs. They were able to mention two or more signs of STIs in men and women and at least one location where treatment of STIs is offered. Knowledge of the means of transmission was inadequate, however, with many teachers expressing their belief that mosquitoes can transmit the disease.

Lessons Learned

Implementation of the program has revealed a number of challenges and yielded a variety of lessons.

Training and Support

Staff and teachers associated with the program identified the need to strengthen training and to provide adequate support for teachers after they begin implementing the program. To meet this challenge, the program has developed training materials that cover didactic strategies (such as lesson planning). Other steps could include establishment of local teacher resource centers that could provide ongoing refresher training and inclusion of PEAS training in existing pre- and in-service training programs.

Student Participation

Program implementers and teachers interviewed indicated that while their students' level of interest and intensity of participation was high, access to and participation in PEAS activities and classes could be improved. A pressing need exists to develop strategies to ensure that all students can attend PEAS classes.

The challenge of increasing access to PEAS teaching is being met by teacher training, which is increasing the number of teachers equipped to deliver the program. Introduction of a peer education component is also increasing student participation and students' sense of ownership of the program. Scope exists to improve student involvement by collaborating with adolescent education centers.

Partnerships

Although significant progress has been made in forging partnerships with both community-based stakeholders and development partners, both the PEAS manager and program implementers believe the program would benefit from further advocacy and partnership-building efforts. In particular, there is a need to ensure that there is consistency between the program's objectives and materials on the one hand and the information that is shared in students' homes on the other.

Parental and community support for PEAS is currently sought through advocacy and parent-teacher meetings. Greater efforts are needed to put in place a mechanism through which the parents of secondary-school students, as well as the parents of younger children, can provide feedback on PEAS and actively contribute to achieving its objectives.

Myths and Prejudices

Myths about and prejudices against people living with HIV/AIDS are deeply entrenched in the Dominican Republic. The evaluation survey showed that many young people believe that HIV/AIDS can be transmitted by mosquito bites, by touching infected people, by sharing kitchen utensils with infected people, or by sharing a toilet with an infected person (see table 1.3).

PEAS objectives, materials, and methods seek to combat such beliefs. Ongoing modification of the program seeks to help it better address myths that govern the sexual behavior of students and teachers, as well as community attitudes toward sex, HIV, and other STIs.

Management and Implementation

Various obstacles confront those responsible for the day-to-day management and implementation of the program and longer-term planning. Vertical information flows are weak: a strategic action plan exists, but the big picture is not shared with those who implement the program.

Regional- and district-level action plans are needed to help program implementers and teachers achieve the objectives set out by the national-level strategic action plan. School-based work plans and lesson plans are needed to help program implementers and teachers set and achieve student participation targets and cover topics laid out in the program materials.

Monitoring and Evaluation

Like many HIV/AIDS education programs worldwide, PEAS does not have an operational monitoring and evaluation (M&E) system. Many schools are not implementing PEAS activities. In those that do, teachers gauge program impact in an ad hoc manner. A change in students' attitudes regarding HIV/AIDS, for example, is assessed by the teacher, who simply talks to them, without recording how their behavior changed.

The Department of Counseling and Psychology of SEE complemented the strategic plan with a strategy detailing how M&E findings should be disseminated to stakeholders and describing follow-up procedures. This strategy holds considerable promise for providing timely and necessary information about the program. Lack of funding, however, may prevent it from being implemented.

Conclusion

The PEAS program shows how a curriculum-based approach used in formal school settings can deliver HIV/AIDS education to a large proportion

(73 percent) of a country's secondary-school students. Implementation of the program varies widely across schools, suggesting that merely training teachers in HIV/AIDS curricula is not enough: program officials must ensure that teaching is monitored and teachers are able to access support, receive ongoing training, and provide input into program development.

Annex 1.1

PEAS Attainment of Impact Benchmarks

BENCHMARK	ATTAINMENT/COMMENTS
1. Identifies and focuses on specific sexual health goals	✓ Program focuses on preventing STIs and HIV/AIDS, as well as reducing the risk of teenage pregnancy.
2. Focuses narrowly on specific behaviors that lead to sexual health goals	✓ Changes in adolescent sexual behavior are major objective of program.
3. Identifies and focuses on sexual psychosocial risk and protective factors that are highly related to each of these behaviors	✓ Program provides instruction on sexual psychosocial risk behaviors, particularly with regard to STIs and HIV/AIDS.
4. Implements multiple activities to change each of the selected risk and protective factors	✓ Program uses a variety of methods, including lectures, case analyses, group discussions, experience sharing, and audio-visual presentations.
5. Actively involves youth by creating a safe social environment	Partial. Activities take place under the supervision of teachers. Peer education has yet to be fully implemented.
6. Employs a variety of teaching methods designed to involve participants and have them personalize the information	✓ Formal class-based instruction is combined with participatory child-led activities.
7. Conveys clear message about sexual activity and condom or contraceptive use and continually reinforces that message	✓ Program promotes both sexual abstinence and condom use.
8. Includes effective curricula and activities appropriate to the age, sexual experience, and culture of participating students	✓ Activities are integrated into national secondary-school curriculum. Education is designed for specific grade/age groups, becoming increasingly complex and dealing more with HIV/AIDS in upper grades. Program designed on the basis of staff experience with and knowledge gained about youth in the Dominican Republic.
9. Increases knowledge by providing basic, accurate information about the risks of teen sexual activity and methods of avoiding intercourse or using protection against pregnancy and STIs.	✓ Information provided by program is based on national and international research.
10. Uses some of the same strategies to change perceptions of peer values, to recognize peer pressure to have sex, and to address that pressure	Partial. See benchmark 5.
11. Identifies specific situations that might lead to sex, unwanted sex, or unprotected sex and identifies methods of avoiding those situations or getting out of them	✓ Curriculum includes case studies, role-play, and dramatizations that encourage participants to develop problem-solving skills.
12. Provides modeling of and practice with communication, negotiation, and refusal skills to improve both skills and self-efficacy in using those skills	Partial. Although program stresses importance of negotiating skills, its focus is on imparting knowledge rather than building these skills.

Annex 1.2

Program Contacts

Cristina Molina/Arisa Hernández (Program Coordinators)
Sexual Affective Education Program (PEAS)
Avenida Maximo Gomez. Numero 18. Santo Domingo, Dominican Republic.
Postal Address: Apartado Postal 1481, Santo Domingo, Republica
Dominicana.
Tel: (809) 688 9700 ext. 2120-2124
Fax: (809) 689 8688 or (809) 682 0788

Notes

1. The survey was administered during the last phase of teacher training. The impact of the program on teachers could thus not be measured.

2. The LQAS method was initially developed in the 1920s for quality control of industrial production. In the mid-1980s the methodology was adapted and applied to the field of public health. Since then it has been used to develop baseline studies and to monitor and evaluate public health programs in Africa, Asia, Eastern Europe, and Latin America. In health systems the "lot" is a certain control area of a health program, such as a supervision area. The LQAS method uses small sizes of random samples to precisely and quickly identify the priorities within a supervision area and across several supervision areas in a certain geographical area.

3. The training was based on two publications, *Evaluation of Community Health Programs, Manual and Workbook for the Participant: Use of LQAS for Surveys* and *Regular Monitoring and Evaluation of Community Health Programs Facilitator Guide: Using the LQAS for Surveys and Regular Monitoring.*

4. The data-collection methodology consisted of two self-administered questionnaires, one for students, the other for teachers. The questionnaires reflected the indicators selected by the teaching team working under SEE/COPRESIDA and a national consultant hired by COPRESIDA. The questionnaires were reviewed and improved following consultation with technical staff of the teaching department of SEE/COPRESIDA. They were tested with students and teachers of the Enedina Puello Renvil School (Liceo Madre Vieja Sur) located in San Cristóbal province, which was not selected in the study sample.

References

SEE. 2006. PEAS Training Statistics 2001/2005. PEAS Program, Santa Domingo, Dominican Republic.

USAID (U.S. Agency for International Development). 2002. *AIDS in the Dominican Republic.* Washington, DC.

World Bank. 2000. *Issues and Options*. Caribbean Group for Cooperation in Economic Development, Washington, DC.

World Bank/COPRESIDA. 2004a. *Dominican Republic HIV/AIDS Prevention and Control Project: Initial Results*. Washington, DC.

———. 2004b. *LQAS Report on the PEAS Program, Dominican Republic*. Washington, DC.

The Rapid Results Initiative at a Glance

Description: Rapid implementation of school-based extracurricular HIV prevention activities yielding results in just 100 days.

Number of participants: More than 40,000 students in 48 schools, including all junior and secondary schools in *zoba* (province) Maekel (31 schools in the *zoba*) and 17 junior and secondary schools in other *zobas* (15 percent of all such schools).

Coverage: Four of Eritrea's six *zobas*: Anseba, Gash-Barka, Maekel, and Northern Red Sea.

Target groups: Students attending public junior high schools (ages 12–15) and secondary schools (ages 16–18). Secondary target population includes parents, teachers, supervisors, school administration, and Education Office staff.

Components: Structural organization; orientation for teachers, students, parents, and other stakeholders; material development and life-skills training; peer education and extracurricular club activities; assessment and evaluation.

Establishment and duration: Begun in 2000; pilot phase took place in Asmara, in *zoba* Maekel, before program expanded. Lessons learned have been incorporated into the life skills curriculum now taught in all junior and secondary schools.

Management: Zoba Ministry of Education offices.

Cost: Implementing teachers received an allowance of about $3 twice a week. Participating students received refreshments costing about $0.65 twice a week. Other expenses included the costs of development; transportation; preparation and printing of manuals, brochures, magazines, and documenting activities (video, photographs, and so forth); training; competitions; and support to school health clubs.

The Rapid Results Initiative, Eritrea

The scale and complexity of the issues surrounding HIV/AIDS present policy makers, planners, and implementers with enormous challenges. The magnitude of the task often means that considerable time and energy are spent working on strategy, policy, and curricular development while little ends up being done on the ground to promote positive behavior in schools.

Recognizing the need to respond quickly to the epidemic, the Eritrean government employed methods developed in the business world to identify prevention activities that would yield results in just 100 days. School-based prevention of HIV was identified as being particularly suitable for such an approach and became a part of Eritrea's Rapid Results Initiative (RRI). RRI is an example of how the will and determination of committed personnel can make a difference in the shortest of time frames.

Description

The RRI program aimed to reduce the transmission of HIV among youth and mitigate the impact of HIV/AIDS by equipping young people with the necessary knowledge and skills to protect themselves from infection. It also sought to enable young people to become behavior change agents, especially among peers and within the general community.

The Ministry of Education developed the program in collaboration with Robert H. Schaffer and Associates (RHS&A), an independent consulting firm and the developer of RRI.[1] The *zoba* offices of the Ministry of Education implemented the program in Eritrea.[2] The ministry was also responsible for producing program materials, disseminating information on the program,

Mussie Habte Ghebretinsae, consultant, conducted the interviews and collected the data for this chapter. Kiflay Andemichael and Negusse Maekele, of the RRI Program, provided support, encouragement, and assistance.

training teachers and peer educators, and conducting ongoing monitoring and evaluation (M&E) of the program.

The RRI program was implemented in collaboration with a number of key national partners. These included the Ministry of Health, which provided technical and training support, and the Ministry of Information, which provided media support to the program. *Zoba* administration and regional assemblies facilitated community mobilization and provided general support; the HIV/AIDS, Malaria, STDs, and Tuberculosis (HAMSET) Project Management Unit mobilized resources and provided technical assistance.[3]

Rationale and History

To date the prevalence of HIV in Eritrea has been comparatively low: the Ministry of Health estimated the national adult prevalence at 2.4 percent in 2004. Having observed the impact of the epidemic in other countries, however, the government has made it a national imperative to ensure that prevalence does not increase and, if possible, declines.

In response to this imperative, policy makers adopted an approach from the business world, RRI. The hope was that the program could jump-start activities in the education sector, through well-planned activities that would achieve meaningful and measurable results within a short period of time (box 2.1). The expectation was that the program would start small and then expand, taking into account lessons learned along the way.

In collaboration with RHS&A, the Ministry of Health initiated the program at a launch attended by all sectors of society, including members of the national government, various line ministries, local government, and civil society. Those attending were invited to identify areas in which work could commence, with the expectation of eliciting change and improvement with respect to HIV prevention within 100 days. Participants then voted on the six most-promising areas, which included the following:

- School-based establishment of behavior change for prevention of HIV

- Establishment of voluntary counseling and testing

- Faith-based home care for people living with HIV/AIDS

- Reduction of needle injuries in hospitals

- Increased condom use among commercial sex workers

- Improved prevention of HIV among truck drivers.

A school-based program was the most popular choice because young people were perceived as the group at greatest risk of infection, and schools

---

Box 2.1: The Rapid Results Initiative

Companies and countries often delay roll-out of large-scale programs because of inadequate implementation capacity. RRI seeks to achieve results that appear beyond reach within very short periods—achievements that inspire others to commit themselves to achieving the same results. Results are achieved through the program's ability to strengthen three critical "capacity levers."

Harnessing the capacity of leaders to challenge and motivate. Breaking results down into 100-day building blocks allows senior people at various levels of government to challenge and motivate teams to achieve superior results.

Empowering local agents and holding them accountable. People respond to a challenge, particularly when it involves a real impact on their lives. Most worthwhile results do not come neatly aligned with governmental units. Rather, they require the collaboration of multiple players in diverse institutions, often spanning several sectors. By focusing on single results for which they feel jointly accountable, people from different organizations are able to transcend some of the typical organizational turf issues. The 100-day implementation cycle provides fast and frequent opportunities for reinforcing necessary attitudes, skills, and behaviors. With each phase, confidence is built at the leadership and local levels. As results are achieved, capacity for implementation and change is strengthened.

Focusing on the approach rather than the content. RRI seeks to channel human and financial resources to achieve results. The approach does not in any way dictate the content of a program, which was determined by the government, which drew on national and international expertise. RHS&A introduced Eritreans to the RRI approach and helped the government translate its ideas and inputs into results.

---

were believed to be among the best places to shape young people's life-long values and behaviors.

Before adopting RRI, members of the Ministry of Education underwent training in life-skills education provided by the United Nations Children's Fund (UNICEF). RRI trainers used the expertise of these staff to establish phase I of an RRI school-based life-skills education program for 100 boys and 100 girls in each of six secondary schools in Eritrea's capital, Asmara (*zoba* Maekel). The schools chosen demonstrated strong leadership and enthusiasm for HIV prevention and life-skills activities. Even as the first phase of RRI was taking place, teachers in other schools were being trained for phase 2 (figure 2.1).

Aims and Objectives

The RRI program tackled HIV prevention in children and youth by teaching them about sex and sexuality. It is based on the idea that knowledge alone is not enough; there is a need to develop life skills so that knowledge can be translated into actions that result in more responsible, healthier behaviors.

Figure 2.1: Timeline of RRI Development

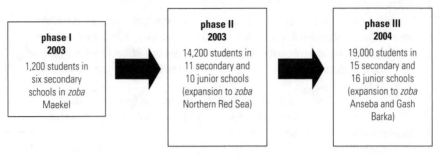

Source: Authors.

The main aim of the program was to reduce the transmission of HIV among youth and mitigate the impact of HIV/AIDS by equipping young people with the knowledge and skills they need to protect themselves from infection and to help others by becoming behavior change agents, especially among their peers and within the general community.

The program included both science-based information about HIV/AIDS (causes, means of transmission, and so forth) and information about human factors affecting the epidemic (cultural values, risky behaviors, stereotypes, denial, stigma). It sought to equip students with the necessary knowledge and skills to achieve the following:

- Delay the age of sexual initiation.

- Avoid HIV infection.

- Become behavior change agents in their communities.

- Help people who are already infected with HIV and teach them how to live positively.

- Stop denial, stigma, and discrimination.

- Consider voluntary counseling and testing.

In addition to addressing risky behavior related to sex, RRI helped students avoid other practices that put them at risk, including the following:

- Cultural practices, such as female genital mutilation

- Traditional healing practices, such as bloodletting

- Use of unsterilized sharp instruments

- Mother-to-child transmission and unsafe blood transfusions.

The program's activities aimed to:

- develop behavior change communication skills

- enhance self-awareness and self-esteem and build confidence

- provide guidance on relationships

- develop negotiation skills

- improve skills to make informed decisions

- develop problem-solving skills

- provide guidance on avoiding risks

- support values clarification

- resist peer pressure from negative influences

- say "no" to sex

- cope with emotions and stress

- show empathy and sympathy

- combat gender stereotypes.

Strategies

RRI sought to achieve its objectives through a range of strategies:

- Conducting peer-led education sessions under the supervision of trained teachers delivered to groups of students within schools

- Targeting the school community by including HIV prevention activities in extracurricular activities

- Reaching out to the wider community through mass media broadcasts, general knowledge contests, music and drama shows, broadcasts, and other means

- Providing students with alternatives to risky behavior by allocating more resources to sports, music facilities, and other school-based activities.

Target Groups

RRI's primary target group was students in public junior high schools (ages 12–15) and secondary schools (ages 16–18). Its secondary target audience was members of the school community (parents, teachers, supervisors, school administration staff, and Education Office staff).

Components

The RRI program included five components:

- Structural organization

- Orientation for teachers, students, parents, and other stakeholders

- Material development and life-skills training

- Peer education and extracurricular club activities

- Assessment and evaluation

    Each of these components is described in the following section.

Implementation

Structural Organization

The structural organization component of the program took place soon after the program was launched. The main purpose was to guide the leadership and delineate roles and responsibilities of all individuals involved in running the program at the *zoba* and school levels (figure 2.2). The strategic leader and the program coach disseminated information about the management of program activities to team leaders, pedagogical heads, work teams (implementers), and peer educators. Supervisors and school administrators also attended this one-day training session.

Training and Orientation

Because RRI draws heavily on community support, it included a component dedicated to introducing the goals and objectives of the program to everyone involved in it. This component took place at the *zoba* level at the start of each new phase of the program.

   During a one-day session, the strategic leader and the program coaches introduced the program to all concerned implementing bodies and explained the main goals and objectives of the program. Orientation was given to teachers that delivered the program (team leaders and work teams), peer educators, parent representatives of the parent-teacher association (PTA), school administrators, and officials and representatives of other key stakeholders (such as the Ministry of Health and NGOs). The session also aimed to raise awareness on the coordination and management structure of the program at the school level. Gaining support from all members of the meeting was

Figure 2.2: Organizational Structure of the Rapid Response Initiative

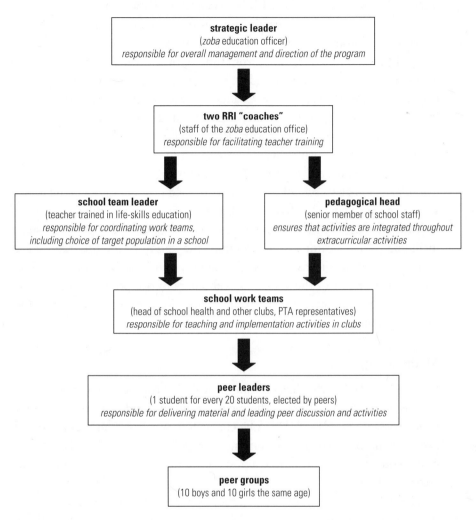

Source: Authors.

crucial. Teachers initially recruited to the program were trained in life skills and active in the development of life skills–based education materials. In later phases teachers chosen were those who showed interest in working with young people and who were competent at and active in organizing and leading activities in their schools.

Following the orientation workshop, training of teachers (including team leaders and work teams), peer educators, and others, including head teachers and supervisors, was carried out over a two-week period. Training was delivered by the strategic leader; the program coaches; health professionals; teachers trained in life skills; and resource people, including people living with AIDS. The main aim of training was to introduce the training manuals to teachers and peer educators; train them in life skills; and familiarize them with participatory methodologies (such as discussions, games, drama, role-plays, and case studies) used in program activities. Training was also provided on the roles and responsibilities of facilitators, case study–based activities, and asking questions to assess attitudes.

In addition to initial training, from time to time during each phase, work teams and peer educators received ongoing training. These sessions updated teachers and peer educators on changes in the program, enhancing their knowledge of life skills and participatory teaching-learning approaches.

Once each phase of RRI began, RRI coaches and school team leaders trained school work teams over the weekend in the topics in the resource manual to be delivered to students the following week. During the week (Monday–Thursday), school team leaders trained peer educators in the topics so that the peer educators could facilitate similar sessions on Friday.

Twice during each phase, meetings were organized for program staff, including peer educators, to discuss implementation of the program, share good practices and ideas, discuss difficulties, and look for solutions. The active involvement of the various stakeholders in the program was consistent with and supported the active, participatory learning approach of the RRI program.

Methodology

Until 2005 HIV/AIDS education was provided during science in junior high schools and during biology at the secondary level. English classes also contained passages on HIV/AIDS. The curriculum was based on the traditional pedagogical approach of transmitting knowledge. In 2005 life skills–based health education was introduced as a subject in upper elementary, junior, and secondary schools.

The RRI program used an extracurricular approach to provide life skills–based education on HIV/AIDS. Peer-led sessions were held for about one and a half to two hours every Friday afternoon, when school ends early. As the program was carried out outside of regular school hours, gaining the support of the community was important; students need the permission of their parents or caregivers to stay at school to take part in these activities.

Peer educators, elected by their classmates and supervised by trained teachers, led groups of 20 students. The peer educators were students who were liked and respected by other students; they tended to be influential opinion leaders. Teachers were on hand to help, but they were not present during sessions, in order to allow students to speak with less inhibition. Reasons for the use of peer educators included the following:

- Peer educators were believed to have more influence than adults on young people.

- Young people listen and discuss matters openly with their peers.

- Peer educators can easily identify and understand the needs of young people.

- Using peer educators makes the learning environment friendlier.

A range of pedagogical approaches supported the RRI program. Teaching and learning were meant to be active, participatory, and relevant to the daily lives of students. A safe environment is important when discussing sensitive topics such as sexuality. Participatory methodologies—dramas, role-plays, case studies, debates—were used to deliver materials. After discussing the materials with peer leaders, different groups presented their understanding of materials to other groups at their school.

Most sessions were taught in mixed groups. Some issues—such as gender roles and sexuality, gender stereotypes and expectations, development of secondary sexual characteristics, feelings and emotions that arise during puberty—were addressed in single-sex groups.

Implementers ranked activities in order of frequency of use as follows:

1. Introduction to the core elements of life skills

2. "My important values" versus "My behavior"

3. Gender stereotypes and expectations

4. Decision-making exercises

5. Peer pressure

6. Group discussions on gender and cultural issues

7. How do you feel about AIDS?

8. Case studies, dramas, questions and answers

9. Games

10. Role-playing

11. Debates and general knowledge competitions

12. Songs

13. Video shows

14. Sports activities

15. Distribution of reading material, such as pamphlets

16. Art exhibitions

> Group discussions, games, role-playing, drama and songs are thought to be more effective because these activities make students active and allow them to participate directly.
>
> Activities which are less participatory such as art exhibitions and distribution of pamphlets are less effective as they have less chance for the direct involvement of students.
>
> *RRI Implementers, zoba Maekel*

HIV prevention education and activities were also included in schools' extracurricular clubs, such as the drama club, the debating club, and the quiz club. These activities enabled messages to reach beyond the school gates to the wider community. For example, students in music and drama clubs produced songs and scripts for street theater. They produced art exhibitions for World AIDS Day. People from outside the school—including representatives from the Ministry of Health, people living with HIV/AIDS, and members of local music and drama clubs—were regularly invited to join the peer-led sessions.

> Community support is vital to program success and effectiveness. The children are from the community and they must be encouraged by the community to join the program. Involving the community in assessing the needs and behavior of youth and keeping them informed of the planned interventions makes them support and advocate for the program.
>
> *RRI Implementers, zoba Maekel*

Materials

RRI drew on a range of sources to produce the teaching manuals and materials developed. In particular, it drew on the expertise of the Information, Communication, and Education Department of the Ministry of Health, which pioneered the implementation of behavior change communication in Eritrea. RRI also drew on life skills materials produced by UNICEF.

The most important materials used by teachers and peer educators were those included in the *HIV/AIDS Life Skills Training Manual* developed by the *zoba* Education Office. Topics covered included the following:

- Decision-making skills

- Risk-assessment skills

- Gender stereotypes

- Values

- Influences (particularly peer pressure)

- Problem-solving skills

- Communication skills

- Coping with stress and emotions.

Production of the training manuals was a continuous process, with fresh editions prepared for each new phase of the program. New editions took into account the aims and objectives of the phase as well as the lessons learned during the previous phase. Manuals also took students' knowledge of HIV (assessed through preprogram surveys) into account. For example, as the program was expanded from secondary schools to junior high schools, it was important to ensure that the delivery of materials was age appropriate. At the junior high level, activities focus on abstinence messages. At the secondary level, activities focus on Abstinence, Being faithful, and Condom use (ABC).

Peer educators received activity sheets to help them conduct activities with their groups (box 2.2). Both teachers and peer educators were given informative brochures and magazines to share with community members and peers.

In addition to the training manual, RRI developed a manual for use within schools. It included age-appropriate activities such as case studies, dramas, games, group discussions, and role-plays.

Box 2.2: Sample Activity: Transmission and Prevention of HIV

Objective: To explain how HIV is transmitted and prevented
Time: 40 minutes
Instruction: Students are divided into groups to read and discuss a case study and then answer questions
Materials: Copies of the following case study:

> *Rahel is a 16-year-old girl who lives with her aunt. She has had several unprotected sexual encounters. Last week she attended a seminar organized by the health club at school about ways HIV is transmitted and prevented. Since then she has started to worry about her situation.*

Questions: Students are asked to answer the following questions and present their answers to the class for further discussion:

1. Why do you think Rahel started to worry?
2. If you were Rahel, what would you do?
3. What advice would you give Rahel?

Learning: After students present their answers, the activity is concluded by presenting the following learning points:

- HIV, the virus that causes AIDS, is transmitted through unprotected sexual contacts with infected people; contact with infected blood; use of unsterilized instruments, such as syringes, needles, and razor blades; and during birth, when it is transmitted from infected mothers to their babies.
- Abstinence and avoidance of unprotected contact with blood-contaminated objects is the best way to avoid HIV infection.

> It's very important that materials are personally relevant to students. They should deal with the special challenges the students are facing, work with their experience and help them solve their own problems. If materials aren't relevant to students they will lose interest, will not "buy into" the program and it will be a failure.
>
> *RRI Implementers, zoba Maekel*

Brochures and magazines were developed for use by the whole community, including teachers, students, parents, and the general public. These materials include information about both HIV/AIDS and the RRI program.

Monitoring and Management

Monitoring and management mechanisms had to evolve to keep pace with the expansion of activities to maintain quality. In phase I two coaches were able to manage six school team leaders and administer all activities. It was quickly realized that such a structure would not be sufficient to manage phases II and III, which saw a large increase in the number of schools, teachers, and students.

Rather than simply recruit more coaches, the *zoba* education officer decided to make RRI a priority for all management staff of the *zoba* education office. All school inspectors were included in RRI training, and monitoring of RRI activities was made a standard component of inspection activities. This decision made RRI a "horizontal" program, fully integrated into the daily work of the *zoba* Ministry of Education, rather than a "vertical" program demanding the recruitment of special staff and new offices. New systems were also set up to ensure that financial disbursements to schools occurred quickly and smoothly.

A core feature of the RRI was the process of monitoring, which began before program implementation and followed the completion of each phase. The main purpose was to identify the needs of beneficiaries; study factors likely to hinder or promote implementation of the program; identify concerns of the wider community; note strong and weak points of the program; seek early remedies for drawbacks and conflicts; document good practices; assess attitudinal and behavioral changes; and promote accountability.

While program activities were running, supervisors conducted periodic inspections. A day for evaluation, involving all individuals involved in the program as well as other stakeholders, was held at the end of each phase to assess whether the work plan was properly implemented; identify program achievements (increased knowledge and skills and changed attitudes and behavior); assess the work done by team leaders, work teams, supervisors, teachers, peer educators, and PTAs; and consider ways forward. Students were not graded on their performance, which was assessed only informally.

Partnerships

RRI depended on the cooperation of many different partners for its success. All partners played important roles (table 2.1).

Costs

Full costing information for the program is not available. Implementing teachers received an allowance of about $3 twice a week. The total allowances provided per teacher per phase came to about $86. Participating students received refreshments costing about $0.65 twice a week (about $19 per student per phase). Other costs incurred during the program included the costs of transportation; development, preparation, and printing of manuals and other materials; training; running competitions; and documenting activities (video, photographs).

Evaluation

The RRI produced measurable results during each phase in a very short period. The program greatly expanded its coverage during each phase, reaching about 40,000 students, teachers, supervisors, school administrators, Education Office staff, and community members.

An important aspect of the RRI approach was the setting of locally defined 100-day goals toward which the program aims and against which its success was measured. "Assessment and evaluation" was formally listed as a program component to highlight the importance of its role within the program. Evaluation at the end of each phase of the program was used as the basis of developing the next phase and as a constant measure of the impact of the program on beneficiaries' knowledge, attitudes, and practices as well as success in reaching program objectives. Data collected throughout the evaluation process were used to replicate, scale up, and expand good practices and rectify drawbacks. The manner in which the evaluation process took place—in particular the direct use of feedback from various sources to improve the program—was consistent with and supportive of the overall participatory learning approach of the RRI program.

Table 2.1: Role of Partners in RRI

MINISTRY OF EDUCATION CENTRAL OFFICE	MINISTRY OF HEALTH	MINISTRY OF INFORMATION
Supported program implementation Engaged partners for resource mobilization, program development, and sustainability Assisted with monitoring and evaluation	Provided training in guidance and counseling for teachers and peer educators Provided technical and financial support Supported preparation of materials and evaluation questionnaires Assisted with program implementation, monitoring, and evaluation	Broadcast general knowledge and debating contests, dramas, and sports activities on radio and television

Source: Author.

Impact on Students

Evaluation of the program's impact on target beneficiaries occurred before the program was initiated and at the end of each of its three phases. The preprogram needs assessment was conducted in about 30 target schools and involved students who would not participate in the intervention. The evaluations carried out at the end of each phase were conducted on a randomly selected one-third of program beneficiaries in all target schools within that phase (about 65 in phase 1, 4,730 in phase 2, and 6,330 in phase 3).

Evaluations were conducted using questions extracted from a Tigrinya-language version of the "International Behavior Survey Learners' Questionnaire," obtained from the Eritrean Ministry of Health National HIV/AIDS Unit. Questions asked during pre- and postinterventions included the following:

- Have you ever had sexual intercourse?
- If so, at what age did you start?
- Did you or your partner use a condom?
- If yes, who suggested using a condom, you or your partner?
- If no, why didn't you or your partner use a condom?
- Have you ever heard of a disease that spreads through sexual intercourse?
- Have you ever heard of HIV or AIDS?
- If yes, what causes it?
- How does it spread and how can one prevent it?
- Do you know anyone who is infected with HIV or anyone who has died of AIDS?

ZOBA ADMINISTRATION AND REGIONAL ASSEMBLY	HAMSET PROJECT MANAGEMENT UNIT	RELIGIOUS LEADERS	PTA
Sensitized and coordinated stakeholders	Assisted with program coordination and resource mobilization	Provided advocacy for the program	Provided advocacy for the program
Provided technical and financial support	Provided technical and financial support	Encouraged student participation	Sensitized parents about the program
Mobilized communities	Supervised, monitored, and evaluated program implementation		Encouraged student participation
Assisted with monitoring and evaluation			

- Can a person get HIV from a mosquito bite?

- Can people protect themselves from AIDS by abstaining from sex?

- Can you tell who is infected with HIV simply by looking at people?

- If a pregnant woman is infected with HIV, do you think she could also transmit the virus to her baby? Why?

- Where do people get tested for HIV?

- Have you ever had an HIV test? If yes, did you do so voluntarily?

- Would you be willing to share your result with another person? If so, with whom?

- What would you do if a close friend or relative were infected with HIV?

- If a student is infected with HIV but is not sick, should he or she be allowed to attend school? Why?

The results showed that the program had a measurable impact on both abstinence and condom use (table 2.2).

Evaluation of Implementers

Throughout each phase, implementers were supervised. In phase I supervision was conducted by the two program coaches. As the program was scaled up, supervision became part of the day-to-day activities of *zoba* Education Office inspectors.

Teachers and peer educators responded to questionnaires about the program's process. Questions asked included the following:

- How was the participation of students and teachers?

- What was the role of peer educators? Were peer educators helpful?

Table 2.2: Impact of RRI on Students

PHASE I	PHASE II	PHASE III
Among students 16–18 who participated in the program, 90 percent reported that they abstained from sex. Three percent reported engaging in safe sex (using condoms).	In junior schools, 98 percent of students reported abstaining from sex. The number of students 16–18 years reporting that they abstained from sex rose to 98 percent. Two percent reported engaging in safe sex (using condoms).	In junior schools, 100 percent of students reported that they abstained from sex. The number of students 16–18 years reporting that they abstained from sex rose to 99 percent. One percent of students reported engaging in safe sex (using condoms).

Source: RRI program.

- What was parents' attitude toward the program?
- What were the positive aspects of the program?
- What changes would you like to see to the program?
- How did you benefit from this program?
- Were there any challenges to the implementation of activities?

Lessons Learned

RRI has consistently built on the results of its assessments and evaluations to improve the program. At each phase it has tried to convert the challenges into lessons learned for the next phase. The issues documented here are based on interviews with program managers and implementers.

Commitment

RRI's expectation that results would be generated within just 100 days demanded enormous political commitment at the highest level to counteract inertia and the tendency of government bureaucracy to respond to challenges slowly. Reflecting on the program, Eritrea's minister of education described RRI as "a new movement." His authority, together with that of the minister of health, was essential to ensure that all concerned with the program ensured that delays in implementation were minimized and bottlenecks not allowed to develop. At the *zoba* level, the strong and dynamic leadership of the education officer was essential to ensure the commitment of staff, the swift resolution of problems, and the rapid initiation of new structures and systems needed to support activities. The commitment of both national and regional leaders has motivated staff associated with the program to implement it with zeal.

Management

Program leaders took the need to achieve results within 100 days very seriously. To do so, the management structure had to be strong enough to provide clear guidance on the development of the program as it expanded over the three phases. Constant evolution of program management was demanded, particularly as activities were expanded. This meant moving from having two coaches in phase I to making RRI a priority for all management staff of the *zoba* Education Office. New systems were implemented to ensure that financial disbursements to schools occurred quickly and smoothly. Staff who were not achieving desired outputs were replaced.

> There are many spices that you have to put into the dish. The main ingredients are committed coaches and life-skills teachers.
>
> The main challenges in managing people involved in RRI is to ask "Who is supporting?," "Who is opposing?," "Who is lagging behind?," "Who is undermining the achievement of results?"
>
> *RRI Strategic Leader, zoba Maekel*

Communication

Excellent public relations were needed to ensure that all students, teachers, communities, and other stakeholders were fully informed about the program as quickly as possible. To do so, the program used radio and television to publicize activities and produced many brochures and magazines about the program.

> Opposition comes from lack of understanding. A major priority of teams was to overcome lack of knowledge.
>
> *RRI Strategic Leader, zoba Maekel*

Constant Assessment

Assessment is a necessary feature of any project to measure success and address shortcomings. It was particularly important for RRI, because the program was constantly expanding. That said, the fact that RRI was such a short-term project made evaluation difficult.

Discussions following each phrase took into account the results of the impact assessment for that phase and the responses of peer leaders, teachers, and team leaders. They also addressed the range of practical issues that emerged during implementation. On the basis of these discussions, changes were made, including revision of training manuals.

Conclusions

RRI can be used to jump-start school-based efforts to educate students about HIV/AIDS. Program implementers believe that the program had a positive effect on the in-school teaching-learning process. The active involvement of teachers, students, and community members in implementing, monitoring, and evaluating the program as well as the active and participatory teaching and learning methods used were beneficial.

The success of the program can be attributed to several factors:

- Each phase of the program could be implemented within a 100-day period.

- A strong organization structure was developed and adopted at all levels of program operation.

- Strong advocacy and sensitization workshops garnered support from all stakeholders at all levels of the program.

- Constant assessment and evaluation ensured that the program was able to build on successes and rectify shortcomings at each phase of the program.

- Development of new training and teaching materials at all phases ensured that they were relevant.

- Training at all phases of the program ensured that implementers were able to make good use of the revised materials.

Annex 2.1

RRS Attainment of Impact Benchmarks

BENCHMARK	ATTAINMENT/COMMENTS
1. Identifies and focuses on specific sexual health goals	Partial. While the main focus of the program is HIV prevention, the program includes other elements, such as personal and environmental hygiene, teenage pregnancy, and alcohol and drugs.
2. Focuses narrowly on specific behaviors that lead to sexual health goals	✓ Program focuses on development of life skills to enable promotion of abstinence; strong, effective, and faithful relationships; and use of condoms.
3. Identifies and focuses on sexual psychosocial risk and protective factors that are highly related to each of these behaviors	✓ Program provides information about HIV and equips students with the skills to identify and avoid risk factors.

(*Continues on the following page*)

BENCHMARK	ATTAINMENT/COMMENTS
4. Implements multiple activities to change each of the selected risk and protective factors	✓ Program uses wide range of strategies, including peer educator–led teaching, extracurricular activities, and provision of alternatives to risky behaviors.
5. Actively involves youth by creating a safe social environment	✓ Emphasis on participative teaching by peer educators creates a safe social environment for participation.
6. Employs a variety of teaching methods designed to involve participants and have them personalize the information	✓ A range of participatory teaching methodologies were used by the program.
7. Conveys clear message about sexual activity and condom or contraceptive use and continually reinforces that message	✓ See benchmark 2.
8. Includes effective curricula and activities appropriate to the age, sexual experience, and culture of participating students	✓ Curricula were targeted at junior and secondary-school students. Constant feedback from students and other stakeholders ensured that materials were tailored to the experience and culture of participants.
9. Increases knowledge by providing basic, accurate information about the risks of teen sexual activity and methods of avoiding intercourse or using protection against pregnancy and STIs	✓ Course content was strong and clear. Students learn how to abstain from sex, avoid risk, say no, and use condoms if they do engage in sex.
10. Uses some of the same strategies to change perceptions of peer values, to recognize peer pressure to have sex, and to address that pressure	✓ Peer teaching is key part of program, enabling questions of peer pressure to be met head on.
11. Identifies specific situations that might lead to sex, unwanted sex, or unprotected sex and identifies methods of avoiding those situations or getting out of them	✓ Role-plays, dramas, case studies, and many other participatory methodologies help students identify situations that might lead to sex and learn how to deal with them.
12. Provides modeling of and practice with communication, negotiation, and refusal skills to improve both skills and self-efficacy in using those skills	✓ Life-skills content of curriculum encourages students to learn and use communication, negotiation, and refusal skills.

Source: Authors.

Annex 2.2

Contact Information

Mr. Kiflay Andemichael
Zoba Maekel Education Officer,
Ministry of Education, Zoba Maekel,
PO Box 82,
Asmara, ERITREA
Tel: +291 1 11 91 02

Ms. Nathalie Gons
Management Consultant,
Rapid Results Institute, Inc.
30 Oak St., Stamford, CT 06905
Tel. +1 718 974-4737
www.rapidresults.org

Notes

1. For more information on the approach, see Matta and Ashkenas (2003) and Matta (2005).

2. The program was implemented in four of Eritrea's six *zobas* (provinces).

3. HAMSET is a project aimed at curbing the spread and impact of HIV&AIDS, Malaria, STDs, and Tuberculosis in Eritrea.

References

Matta, N. 2005. "Unleashing Implementation Capacity in Developing Countries." In *Rapid Results! How 100-Day Projects Develop the Capacity for Large-Scale Change*, eds Robert H. Schaffer and Ronald N. Ashkenas, with colleagues. San Francisco: Jossey-Bass.

Matta, N., and Ronald N. Ashkenas. 2003 "Why Good Projects Fail Anyway." *Harvard Business Review*, September. 109–14.

The Integrated Sectorwide HIV/AIDS Preventive Education at a Glance

Number of schools participating: All upper-basic and secondary-school students in The Gambia receive classroom teaching on HIV/AIDS as part of the school curriculum; 160 of 270 upper-basic and senior-secondary schools and 194 of 335 lower-basic schools have peer education programs.

Coverage: Nationwide. Program has trained 4,217 peer educators (53 percent of them girls). In 2003–04, when total enrollment was 238,000 (178,000 at basic level, 60,000 at secondary level), more than 90,000 students were reached with peer education.

Target groups: Children and youth 4–19, teachers, and other school personnel. Education on HIV/AIDS is currently provided only to students in lower- and upper-basic and secondary school. In the future, the program hopes to expand reach to preschool students as well. Secondary target group includes family members of children and youth.

Components: Curriculum-based teaching about HIV, teacher training and orientation on HIV, peer health education, guidance and counseling, establishment of HIV/AIDS clubs, outreach to out-of-school youth, and outreach to the community.

Establishment and duration: Peer education began in 1990. Teacher training began in 1991. HIV/AIDS was integrated into a carrier course in 1992. An HIV/AIDS unit was established within the Department of State for Education in 2002. Peer education was expanded in 2002. A trinational response by The Gambia, Liberia, and Sierra Leone began in 2004.

Role of Department of State for Education: Coordinates all HIV prevention activities, including those led by NGOs.

Role of partners: The Nova Scotia–Gambia Association is involved in implementing peer education program activities.

Chapter 3

Key evaluation results: A survey conducted by Catholic Relief Services in 2003 (one year after the expansion of activities) found that:

- about 85 percent of students had heard of HIV/AIDS;

- students had access to information from a variety of sources;

- 1–3 percent of the student body reported having had one-on-one discussions about HIV/AIDS with a peer health educator; and

- 60 percent of teachers interviewed volunteered information about the presence of HIV/AIDS programs in their schools.

Integrated Sectorwide HIV/AIDS Preventive Education, The Gambia

As HIV/AIDS is becoming more of a development problem rather than an exclusive health issue, children, youth, teachers and education sector personnel (vulnerable groups) will be targeted to slow the spread and progression of the pandemic. HIV/AIDS issues will be taught in all learning institutions to ensure that these institutions are used as effective vehicles to intensify the HIV/AIDS sensitization in communities.

Taken from The Gambia's Education Policy (2004–2015)

Education-sector prevention of HIV/AIDS demands the participation of many different stakeholders, including government, teachers, students, parents, and communities. For the participation of so many different groups to be effective, efforts must be well planned and coordinated to avoid duplication, confusion, and wasted effort. The Gambia's integrated sectorwide HIV/AIDS preventive education program is a unique country-level response to HIV. The program is coordinated by the Department of State for Education (DoSE) and implemented by a range of partners. The Gambia also works with other countries, with the aim of delivering a harmonized, region-specific, and culturally sensitive response. The coordination has enabled a wide range of government agencies and nongovernmental organizations (NGOs) to undertake activities with direction, coherence, and vigor.

Sherif Yunus Hydara, of the Department of State for Education (DoSE), conducted the interviews and collected the data for this chapter. Momodou Sanneh, Director of Basic and Secondary Education, DoSE; Amicoleh Mbaye, HIV/AIDS Focal Point, DoSE; Isatou Ndow, Head, School of Education, Gambia College; Haddy Jammeh, Regional Education Directorate 2, Brikama; Saihou Ceesay, Director, National AIDS Secretariat; Nuha Ceesay, Deputy Director, National AIDS Secretariat; Saidou Jallow, Information, Education, and Communication/Behavior Change Communication Specialist, National AIDS Secretariat; Marian Allen, Principal, St. John's School for the Deaf; Sulayman Njie, Principal, Muslim Senior-Secondary School; Abdoulie Mboge, Deputy Head, Campama Lower-Basic School; and Ansumana Dibba, National Program Coordinator, Nova Scotia-Gambia Association provided support, encouragement, and assistance.

Description

Rationale and History

The Gambia has been addressing HIV/AIDS through the education sector since the late 1980s. In 1991 it established a multisectoral group to develop student texts and teacher guides for basic, upper-basic, and senior-secondary schools. A training manual was developed and two HIV/AIDS teachers trained for each school in the country. Religious and opinion leaders were also trained, to ensure support for the program at the community level.

At the time the materials were introduced, the prevalence of HIV in The Gambia was low, and there was great skepticism regarding the existence of HIV/AIDS. Many believed that HIV/AIDS messages were designed to destroy traditional cultural norms concerning marriage and sexuality rather than to prevent an emerging epidemic. Teachers and parents successfully opposed the teaching of HIV/AIDS in schools. A considerable part of the education sector's response to HIV/AIDS has been to challenge denial concerning the pandemic and to encourage Gambians to recognize the threat it poses.

> Messages are confusing sometimes because when you are taught in school that HIV/AIDS is not curable, you hear from some students arguing that you just need some traditional medicine to cure it.
>
> *Program Student*

In 1992 HIV/AIDS teaching was integrated into a carrier subject, Population and Family Life Education (POP/FLE). The development of POP/FLE as a subject has been supported by the United Nations Family Planning Association (UNFPA) and includes teaching about population, health and the environment, human growth and development, parenthood, vocational awareness, and gender issues. Inclusion of HIV/AIDS in this course has enabled the education sector to break through the silence and denial that often surround HIV/AIDS and ensure that all children in grades 4–12 are educated about the disease.

The Gambia also made early efforts to introduce peer health education. In 1990, with funding from the Canadian International Development Agency (CIDA), the Nova Scotia–Gambia Association (NSGA) conducted a six-week training program in Nova Scotia for 16 students and 3 staff members from St. Peter's Technical High School, in Lamin. The program focused on HIV/AIDS and other STIs, as well as on tobacco, marijuana, and other harmful substances.

During the 1990–91 school year, the St. Peter's team disseminated information to students in a dozen other secondary schools in The Gambia.

Between 1994 and 1996, with funding from Health Canada (Canada's Federal Department of Health), NSGA extended the peer health education program to another 10 senior-secondary schools throughout the country. These teams in turn introduced peer health education in another 16 schools. Activities were sustained at a relatively low level until 2001, when the secretary of state for DoSE, one of the original teachers trained in Canada in 1990, asked NSGA to extend the program throughout the nation's secondary schools. NSGA accepted this challenge and expanded the program, with funding from CIDA (2001–03) and the World Bank (2003–05), through the National AIDS Secretariat (NAS).

In 2001 the HIV/AIDS Rapid Response Project was established, through a $50 million loan from the World Bank. Under the terms of the project, the NAS was created to implement the decisions of the National AIDS Council, a group chaired by the president of The Gambia and made up of secretaries of state, religious leaders, representatives of NGOs, people living with HIV/AIDS, and other stakeholders. In 2002 NAS and DoSE signed a Memorandum of Understanding to establish an HIV/AIDS unit within DoSE. This unit is responsible for coordinating all HIV prevention activities in The Gambia, including both those led by DoSE and those led by NGOs.

With funding from the government of Canada and in cooperation with DoSE, in 2005 NSGA created a new program, Improving Community Health through Youth Development and Leadership. This program enables the 60 school-based peer health education teams (nearly 2,000 trained peer health educators) that have shown the greatest sustainability to work with NSGA's community-based drama troupes to extend the benefits of the program to 100 communities throughout the country.

Since 2004 The Gambia has been part of an interactive network of ministry of education HIV/AIDS "focal points" (ministry officers charged with oversight of the issue) drawn from all 15 francophone, anglophone, and lusophone countries in the Economic Community of West African States (ECOWAS) and Mauritania (box 3.1). The objective of the network is to accelerate the education sector response to HIV/AIDS in the region by:

- creating a framework for sharing information and experiences,

- proposing guidelines and promoting good practices,

- providing information to the Conference of Ministry of Education of ECOWAS and Mauritania on the progress of the education sector response to HIV/AIDS in the region,

- advocating for broad-based commitment and support to the education response to HIV/AIDS,

Box 3.1: Sharing Information within the Region

The Gambia has already moved in the direction of harmonizing regional education sector responses to HIV/AIDS. NSGA's peer health education program has been adopted in Sierra Leone. Sierra Leone's "Sissy Aminata" classroom discussion materials (based on Zimbabwe's "Auntie Stella" materials) were used to prepare The Gambia's "Mam Haddy" materials (a student reader, a teachers' guide, and a peer health educators' guide).

- developing the capacity of focal points, and

- monitoring progress.

Aims, Objectives, and Strategies

The DoSE program aims to enable the education sector to play an important role in stemming the tide of the AIDS pandemic by ensuring that HIV is addressed throughout the sector. The program's objectives are to equip all those associated with the education sector with the information, knowledge, and skills needed to understand and use methods of HIV prevention in their every day lives and to encourage them to educate others about HIV prevention.

Program strategies include the following:

- Developing an education sector response to HIV/AIDS that integrates policy and program responses

- Increasing understanding of HIV/AIDS among all those associated with the education sector

- Including HIV/AIDS throughout sector approaches.

Target Groups

The program plans to target all children and youth 4–19. It is currently providing education to students 7–19 enrolled in lower-basic, upper-basic, and secondary school. Teachers, other education personnel, and DoSE civil servants are also targeted. The secondary target group consists of family members of the primary target group, who are reached through community outreach programs.

Components

The program consists of eight components:

- Curriculum-based teaching about HIV/AIDS

- Training and orientation in HIV/AIDS for teachers

- Sensitization and training of DoSE staff

- Peer health education

- Guidance and counseling

- HIV/AIDS clubs

- Outreach to out-of-school youth

- Outreach to the community

Each of these components is discussed in the next section.

Implementation

Management Structure

The DoSE HIV unit plays two roles. First, it coordinates the work of all stakeholders working in the education sector on HIV/AIDS education. Second, it implements activities such as teacher training, guidance, and counseling.

Implementation of activities across the country is decentralized, with day-to-day responsibility lying with focal points located in each of the country's six regions. At the school level, each institution has an HIV focal point teacher responsible for activities. Focal points are expected to coordinate all HIV/AIDS activities in their schools, including school-based workshops for teachers and extracurricular activities for students. They are also responsible for ensuring that teachers teach the subject effectively.

Most activities occur at a national scale across all schools in the country. Some activities have yet to fully go to scale. NSGA's peer health education activities, for example, have been implemented in 160 of the country's 270 upper-basic and senior-secondary schools (the original project design envisaged reaching only 30–60 schools). In 2005 peer health education was provided in 194 of 335 of the country's lower-basic primary schools, including 102 UNICEF–sponsored girl-friendly schools.

Curriculum-Based Teaching about HIV/AIDS

Education on HIV/AIDS is a module within the POP/FLE course, which is taught to all students in lower-basic, upper-basic, and secondary school. All students are taught POP/FLE for 45 minutes a week in lower-basic school and 60 minutes a week in upper-basic and senior-secondary schools.

Teaching and learning focus mainly on building knowledge about HIV/AIDS. Complementary (co-curricular and extracurricular) activities, such as peer-led activities and sessions with guidance and counseling teachers, focus on skills and attitudes, including learning to say no, to be faithful to one's partner, and to abstain from sex before marriage. Less attention is given to skill building in using condoms correctly and consistently.

Teacher Training and Materials

Teachers are trained by lecturers from the Gambia Teacher Training College. Trainers receive intensive training on the program approach and the use of materials.

Training in HIV education is a requirement for receiving a certificate from the Gambia Teacher Training College. A compulsory course on HIV/AIDS covers the following topics:

- HIV/AIDS and related diseases

- Global impact of HIV/AIDS

- Protecting oneself from HIV/AIDS

- Use of student-centered approaches in HIV/AIDS education

- Counseling on HIV/AIDS

- HIV/AIDS as a developmental issue

- Assessment tools for HIV/AIDS education.

> At The Gambia College, School of Education, we train teachers for lower and secondary school. In order to fight HIV/AIDS, it is necessary and important to train student teachers who will go to the schools with knowledge of HIV prevention. As they are young people, the training will also allow them to have access to information on HIV/AIDS. Teachers are supposed to be role models especially young ones. They can be role models to children and to members of the community.
>
> *Coordinator and Head of The Gambia College, School of Education*

Teachers are trained at both the central and regional levels.
As of 2005 training had been provided to:

- 786 classroom teachers,

- 150 guidance and counseling personnel,

- 150 nonformal instructors,

- 60 instructors at skill and vocational centers,

- 44 early childhood education facilitators,

- 20 special-needs teachers,

- 570 peer health educators, and

- 350 teachers trained by NSGA as teacher-coordinators of the peer health education program.

Teaching about HIV is grade appropriate and builds on the knowledge students acquire in each grade. It includes the provision of clear information about the definition and biology of HIV/AIDS and other STDs, transmission of HIV, prevention of transmission, and the care of people living with HIV/AIDS.

Understanding of school-based HIV prevention has progressed considerably since the development of the POP/FLE curriculum in 1991. Recognizing this, DoSE is in the process of revising and unifying all curricula for life-skills teaching, including the curricula for POP/FLE, guidance and counseling, and teacher training.

DoSE provides teachers with an extensive up-to-date training package to enable them to:

- organize and deliver educational activities and lessons that equip students with the knowledge, skills, and attitudes they need to help prevent the spread of HIV/AIDS

- take care of people affected by the pandemic

- cope with student and teacher absenteeism and illness caused by HIV/AIDS

- provide moral support, counseling, and special attention to children orphaned by HIV/AIDS.

One or more teachers from every school in The Gambia attends a one-week workshop to train them about HIV and to familiarize them with the training manual (described below). Teachers are provided with extensive information about skills-based HIV prevention and familiarized with a range of participatory strategies.

In 2002 DoSE's HIV unit produced a *Training Manual on HIV/AIDS and Education for Teachers and Teacher Trainers*. The manual covers the following topics:

- History and definition of HIV/AIDS

- Causes of HIV/AIDS

- Mode of transmission of HIV/AIDS

- Global and national HIV/AIDS situation

- The National AIDS Secretariat and Control Program

- Prevention of HIV/AIDS

- Impact of HIV/AIDS on the education sector

- Education sector responses to HIV/AIDS

- Care and support for people living with or affected by HIV

- Guidance and counseling on HIV/AIDS

- Voluntary counseling and testing for HIV/AIDS

- Other STIs

- Reducing vulnerability

- Gender dimension.

Teacher training occurs using the *Students' Manual for Population and Family Life Studies.* There are three POP/FLE books for students of different grades: 4–6 (ages 10–13), 7–9 (ages 13–16), and 10–12 (ages 16–18). Teacher guides detailing the aim, teaching process, and assessment of lessons accompany the series.

An important aspect of training is its assumption that the prevention of HIV is the responsibility of everyone in the education sector. Materials do not target students alone; the roles of teachers, teacher unions, parent-teacher associations, and teacher training colleges are also discussed.

> The program aims to provide education sector personnel and clients with the required knowledge, skills and attitudes to protect themselves and to support and care for any of their family members who may be affected by HIV/AIDS.
>
> *DoSE HIV/AIDS and Education Focal Point*

Sensitizing and Training DoSE Staff

DoSE staff attend at least one session on prevention and control of HIV/AIDS and voluntary counseling and testing. This training is provided to ensure that DoSE staff accept and appreciate the presence of the pandemic and participate fully in supporting the program. Sixteen SQAD (Standard and Quality Assurance Directorate) officers and 12 regional education directorate focal points received intensive training on how to coordinate and monitor the activities of teachers who teach HIV prevention.

Peer Health Education

NSGA's nine regional coordinators are in charge of training peer health education in upper-basic and senior-secondary schools (one for each region except the western region, where there are three coordinators). Each coordinator is responsible for organizing training sessions in about 20 schools. Training occurs over the course of a year and addresses both the content of the program and presentation skills. In 2003 NSGA expanded its training base by training two teacher coordinators in each school to train, coach, and monitor peer health educators.

By the end of 2005 NGSA had:

- established peer health education teams in 149 schools and institutions and reached students in another 9 institutions

- trained more than 7,000 peer health educators, of which more than 2,500 had graduated

- reached more than 90,000 students a year.

Within each school NSGA training staff, volunteer medical personnel, and other resource people provide peer health educators (usually 10 boys and 10 girls) with up-to-date information on the major health issues confronting young people. Peer health educators are trained in presentation skills that enable them to reach out to their fellow students, out-of-school youth, and members of their communities. A trained teacher-coordinator facilitates work within the school, ensuring that peer health educators have the support of the school administration and staff; providing coaching, encouragement, and logistical assistance; and monitoring activities for accuracy, quality, and impact. NSGA's peer health education program also has a very active team of peer health educators at Gambia College, many of whom volunteer to become teacher-coordinators of the program in the schools to which they are posted.

The main activity led by peer health educators is delivery, classroom by classroom, of six- to eight-minute dramatic presentations (role-plays, skits, and short dramas) on a range of health topics, including HIV/AIDS, STIs, substance abuse and addiction, tuberculosis, diabetes, malaria, and the establishment of healthy relationships. After the drama presentation, peer health educators engage the audiences in dialogue about the issues raised and follow up with information, problem-solving exercises, role-plays, and other participatory activities. The aim is to encourage audiences to examine the consequences of common health-related actions and behaviors that may put individuals and groups at risk and to adopt behaviors that lead to personal and communal health and well-being. Peer health educators back up their presentations by creating posters and other visual displays on key issues and by inviting guest speakers on health topics to address students at assemblies.

Peer health educators encourage the training of peer education teams in other schools and assist the training of such teams. They also help train their replacements in their school as they approach graduation.

In some schools peer health educators have established teen health centers, where students can come for peer counseling. They also work together with the school guidance counselor. From time to time, peer educators also visit lower-basic schools in their area to deliver messages to students there.

NSGA has produced a manual for peer health educators that covers the following topics:

- Human reproduction

- Puberty

- Conception and pregnancy

- Childbirth

- Infertility

- Urinary tract infections

- STIs (including HIV/AIDS)

- Drug addiction (substance abuse and tobacco)

- Diabetes

- Tuberculosis

- Malaria

- Health relationships (including some teaching on life skills).

Guidance and Counseling

Training in guidance and counseling is provided through workshops led by members of DoSE's guidance and counseling unit. Training has been provided to at least one teacher in more than 90 percent of the country's upper-basic and senior-secondary schools and about half of the country's lower-basic schools.

Working with individuals or groups of children, teachers enable development through understanding and teaching of:

- personal and social development, including life skills, communication skills, and anger management

- educational development, including educational guidance and study skills

- career and vocational development, including career choice, training, and job application skills

- health education development

- gender sensitivity, including gender roles and stereotypes.

In 2003 the guidance and counseling unit of DoSE published a guidance and counseling program training manual. The manual, which is used to train school counselors throughout the country, covers the following topics:

- Behavior modification

- Effective communication skills

- Anger management

- Educational guidance

- Education plans

- Educational options and opportunities

- Career and vocational development

- Career practice skills

- Career training opportunities

- Lifestyles and values

- Peer and reproductive health education

- Gender sensitivity

Women and girls are more vulnerable [to infection] because of their economic status. Traditional values also expose this group to more vulnerability as young girls sometimes marry much older men who are already in polygamous relationships.

DoSE HIV/AIDS and Education Focal Point

HIV/AIDS Clubs

HIV/AIDS clubs in lower-basic and basic-cycle schools have implemented programs in collaboration with the HIV/AIDS unit. These clubs complement the activities led by peer health educator by delivering dramatic presentations to other students about HIV prevention and control and the establishment of healthy relationships. Clubs are also engaged in other activities, such as essay and poster contests. HIV/AIDS clubs have been established in 86 of the country's 480 schools.

Outreach to Out-of-School Youth and the Community

As well as working in and around schools, the NSGA program coordinates outreach to out-of-school youth and the community. Out-of-school youth are reached through a range of organizations, including the Gambian National Youth Council, the Lend-a-Hand Society, Children against AIDS, the Child Protection Alliance, and the Red Cross.

NSGA employs six regional drama troupes, made up of peer educators who recently graduated from high school. These troupes tour the country, giving presentations about HIV/AIDS and other issues. They have reached more than half of all communities. NSGA also produces full-length and short videos, produced in four local languages, which are shown outdoors on large screens. More than 70,000 people have been reached in this way since the program's inception. A weekly radio program is broadcast to reinforce the program's messages.

In 2005 Gambia's National Youth Council, in collaboration with the government and UNICEF, produced a manual designed for use with both in and out-of-school youth entitled "Healthy Relationships for a Better Future: Life Skills Program and Training Manual for Young People in The Gambia." The manual outlines eight sessions, each with a number of participatory activities:

Session 1: Getting Acquainted

Session 2: Understanding Your Body

Session 3: STIs, HIV/AIDS, and Risk-Reduction Behavior

Session 4: Life Skills: Why We Need Them

Session 5: Critical Thinking and Decision-Making Skills

Session 6: Communicating and Relationship Skills

Session 7: Emotion Management Skills

Session 8: Looking at the Future

Student Assessment

Formal assessment occurs through examinations conducted at the end of each term, depending on the school's exam procedures. Quiz, essay, poster, and drama contests are organized for each level, at the end of the term or the end of the year. The contents enhance the capacities of both teachers and students in understanding HIV/AIDS issues and concerns.

Evaluation

DoSE's supervision and inspection unit monitors curricular activities. NSGA coordinators and trainers visit and monitor the progress of peer health education program delivery throughout the country, using a standardized form about program activities. Monitoring and evaluation processes need to be strengthened.

Information about the peer health education activities provided by NGSA was collected in 2003 through a study carried out by Catholic Relief Services. Structured questionnaires were provided to 600 students in grades 7–12 in 11 basic, upper, and senior Catholic secondary schools. The study found that student knowledge of different STIs varied across diseases (table 3.1). It also revealed that students obtain knowledge about HIV/AIDS from a wide range of sources, the most important of which is mass media (table 3.2). School dramas were a significant source of information for many students. Individual conversations with peer health educators were a source of information for just 4 percent of respondents.

Students were found to discuss HIV with a wide range of people (table 3.3). Class and school teachers were found to be students' preferred contacts with whom to discuss HIV. Very few students relied on peer health educators.

While 58.5 percent of students had discussed HIV/AIDS with a friend or classmate, only 29.2 percent had spoken about HIV/AIDS with a peer

Table 3.1: Student Knowledge of Sexually Transmitted Infections

SEXUALLY TRANSMITTED INFECTION	PERCENT
HIV/AIDS	84.5
Gonorrhea	37.9
Syphilis	30.6
Hepatitis	0.2
Chlamydia	0.2

Source: Catholic Relief Services 2003.

Table 3.2: Students' Sources of Information about HIV/AIDS

SOURCE	PERCENT
Gambia AIDS Service	84.3
Television	80.6
Radio	78.7
School drama	56.5
Teacher	46.0
Neighbors or friends	41.5
Student association	35.0
Newspapers, magazines, and other print media	31.5
Formal class	16.5
Street/neighborhood	4.6
Peer health educators	4.0
Health facility workers	3.2
Medical personnel	2.2
Sensitization campaigns and workshops	1.6

Source: Catholic Relief Services 2003.

Table 3.3: People with Whom Students Discuss HIV

PERSON	PERCENT
Teachers	38.3
Friends	37.9
Siblings	27.1
Mother	19.9
Father	15.5
Health personnel	14.4
Peer health educators	1.8

Source: Catholic Relief Services 2003.

health educator. Only 13.5 percent of respondents believed that peer health educators are knowledgeable; 12 percent believed that they are patient, 7 percent that they keep secrets, and 10 percent that they are good listeners.

With 20 peer health educators in a school of 700–2,000 students, their capacity to reach many of their fellow students through one-on-one discussions is limited, especially in a busy urban environment in which many schools run double shifts. The fact that 29.2 percent of students had had a one-on-one discussion with a peer health educator on HIV/AIDS is a sign that the small number of peer health educators is doing a good job in providing one-on-one information to fellow students outside the main drama-based approach.

Lessons Learned

Program Quality

NSGA reports that the sustainability of its program is not uniform (http://www.novascotiagambia.ca). Some schools have demonstrated capacity to sustain the peer health education program on their own; others are incapable of operating such programs or require more assistance to achieve sustainability. About one-third of secondary schools fall into each category.

In schools in which operation of the peer health education program is below standard, NSGA is sending experienced staff and drama troupe members to conduct classroom- by-classroom presentations with members of the school team. Whether such assistance will strengthen management commitment and capacity to improve the delivery of the program in schools remains to be seen. Maintaining and enhancing high-quality implementation of the program will present a considerable challenge when DoSE takes over the running of the program on its own.

Peer Health Educators

The Catholic Relief Services study on perceptions of people living with HIV/AIDS among school children in basic, upper-basic, and secondary schools within the Catholic diocese of Banjul suggests that school drama presentations about HIV/AIDS are an important source of information for many young people. The study also shows that peer health educators' ability to interact with other students as promoters of behavior change is highly limited, with very few students believing that peer health educators were effective in one-to-one situations.

The poor perceptions of performance by peer health educators in one-to-one encounters may reflect a number of causes. It may be that insufficient training has occurred to enable them to act responsibly and effectively in counseling situations. It may also be that it is unreasonable to expect young people to attain performance standards that would be expected of professionals. The number of peer health educators (who make up just only 1–3 percent of the student body) may be too low to sustain counseling. More work needs to be conducted to determine whether these or other factors explain the poor regard in which individual encounters with peer health educators are held.

Teacher Education

The Catholic Relief Services study found that many students viewed their teachers as appropriate and effective people with whom to discuss their behavior and HIV/AIDS. It also found that while the overwhelming majority of teachers had heard about HIV/AIDS and were aware of its modes of transmission and prevention, 70 percent did not know about the use of antiretroviral therapy to prevent mother-to-child transmission of HIV, 94 percent believed that people could be protected from HIV/AIDS by taking antibiotics before having intercourse, and just 60 percent responded spontaneously about the presence of HIV/AIDS programs in their school.

As in many countries, turnover and redeployment of teachers poses a continuous challenge to the provision of HIV/AIDS education in schools. Ongoing teacher training by DoSE's HIV/AIDS unit is essential to respond to the challenge of teacher turnover and to enhance and sustain the capacity of teachers to guide students in their behavior. The program has identified the lack of such support as one of its main challenges and aims to address the problem in the future.

Religious Institutions' Attitude toward Use of Condoms

Many religious leaders in The Gambia feel that abstinence is the best practice for unmarried people, particularly for girls. They believe faithfulness should be absolute after marriage and that the use of condoms should not therefore be necessary. Condom use, according to this view, encourages promiscuity.

DoSE seeks to address this opposition by educating as many different stakeholders as possible, including religious leaders. Achieving progress will be a long-term and demanding activity.

Conclusions

The Gambia had adopted a range of strategies to educate young people about HIV/AIDS. Activities are implemented by a wide variety of partners and supported by sectorwide education and participation of members of DoSE. A concern when many different types of work are being undertaken by many actors is that messages may clash and efforts be duplicated. The Gambia has responded to these concerns by putting in place a system of coordination through DoSE's HIV/AIDS coordination unit, which ensures that all stakeholders act in a concerted fashion so that strengths can be built on and activities synergized.

The work of all stakeholders has been highly effective in challenging denial of HIV and providing students with solid information about the infection. The next challenge is to build on achievements by increasing the quality, coverage, and coordination of life-skills teaching across the country's schools.

Annex 3.1

Integrated Sectorwide HIV/AIDS Preventive Education Attainment of Impact Benchmarks

BENCHMARK	ATTAINMENT/COMMENT
1. Identifies and focuses on specific sexual health goals	Partial. Different activities focus on specific goals to different extents. Some (such as teacher capacity building) focus on transmission and prevention of HIV and on enabling students to take control of their own sexual lives and avoid infection. Others (such as peer health education) include other topics such as smoking and diabetes.
2. Focuses narrowly on specific behaviors that lead to sexual health goals	✓ Program focuses on promotion of abstinence and creation of strong, effective, and faithful relationships. Teaching about condoms is present but not the main focus.
3. Identifies and focuses on sexual psychosocial risk and protective factors that are highly related to each of these behaviors	✓ Program focuses on enabling students to take control of their own sexual lives, particularly by helping them avoid sex and learning to say no.
4. Implements multiple activities to change each of the selected risk and protective factors	✓ Program uses a wide range of strategies, including curriculum based education, school health clubs, peer educators, and outreach to the community.
5. Actively involves youth by creating a safe social environment	✓ Gender- and age-sensitive teaching, use of peer, and other strategies create a safe social environment for participation.
6. Employs a variety of teaching methods designed to involve participants and have them personalize the information	✓ Wide variety of participatory teaching methodologies are used to teach program curriculum.
7. Conveys clear message about sexual activity and condom or contraceptive use and continually reinforces that message	Partial. Students learn principally about abstinence and faithfulness. Program also provides information about condom use, although this is more limited.
8. Includes effective curricula and activities appropriate to the age, sexual experience, and culture of participating students	✓ Curricula and messages are appropriate to the age and circumstances of students.
9. Increases knowledge by providing basic, accurate information about the risks of teen sexual activity and methods of avoiding intercourse or using protection against pregnancy and STIs.	✓ Course content concerning knowledge about HIV is strong and clear.
10. Uses some of the same strategies to change perceptions of peer values, to recognize peer pressure to have sex, and to address that pressure	✓ Use of drama by peers is an effective means of teaching about HIV/AIDS. Peer health educators are less effective in one-to-one counseling situations.
11. Identifies specific situations that might lead to sex, unwanted sex, or unprotected sex and identifies methods of avoiding those situations or getting out of them	✓ Role-play and dramas help students to identify situations that might lead to sex and work through how they can use refusal skills to avoid having sex.
12. Provides modeling of and practice with communication, negotiation, and refusal skills to improve both skills and self-efficacy in using those skills	✓ Life-skills content of curriculum encourages students to learn and use communication, negotiation, and refusal skills.

Source: Authors.

Annex 3.2

Contact Information

Directorate of Basic and Secondary Education
Regional Education Directorate 1
Kanifing, The Gambia
Tel: 00220 4397290

Life Skills Unit
Directorate of Basic and Secondary Education
Willy Thorpe Place Building
Banjul, The Gambia
Tel: 00220 4227621

National Aids Secretariat
7 Clarkson Street
Banjul, The Gambia
Tel: 00220 4223263

Nova Scotia Gambia Association
87 Kairaba Avenue
K.M.C., The Gambia
Tel: 00220 4496927

School of Education
Gambia College
Brikama, The Gambia
Tel: 00220 4483062

A variety of materials is available from the program:
Students' Manual on Population and Family Life Studies, Primary and Higher
Teacher's Certificate Program
The Gambia Population and Family Life Education Pupils' Books, grades 4–6,
7–9, and 10–12
The Gambia Population and Family Life Education Teacher's Guides, grades 4–6,
7– 9, and 10–12
Guidance and Counseling Training Manual
*Training Manual on HIV/AIDS and Education for Teachers and Teacher
Trainers*

To obtain these materials, please contact:
Life Skills Unit
Directorate of Basic and Secondary Education
Willy Thorpe Place Building
Banjul, The Gambia
Tel: +00220 4227621

Reference

CRS (Catholic Relief Services). 2003. *Study on the Perceptions about PLHA among School Children in Upper Basic, Basic Cycle and Secondary Schools within the Catholic Diocese of Banjul.* Banjul, The Gambia.

The School Health Education Program (SHEP) at a Glance

Description: Established national guidelines to ensure consistent implementation of school-based education on HIV prevention by range of stakeholders

Number of schools participating: All schools (basic to senior secondary)

Coverage: Nationwide (138 districts)

Target groups: School-going children aged 4–14 in public basic and junior-secondary schools; secondary target group includes parents and school communities

Components: Establishment of national guidelines to ensure consistent implementation of school-based HIV prevention education; regional and district coordination of stakeholders in the content and delivery of school-based HIV prevention activities; sensitization of parents and school community about program activities; capacity building of various actors to ensure maximum efficiency; and close collaboration of program coordinators with Ministry of Health counterparts at all levels.

Duration: Began in 1992; envisaged as long-term, permanent program

Management: SHEP

Role of Ministry of Education, Science and Sports: HIV/AIDS Secretariat coordinates all HIV/AIDS activities in all departments and agencies under the ministry and offers support

Role of key partners: Donors provide support for funding and technical support for program implementation; NGOs, community-based organizations, and faith-based organizations are involved in program implementation.

Costs: Not available

Key evaluation results: Program has not been evaluated.

The School Health Education Program (SHEP), Ghana

Limited government capacity is often augmented by resources, actions, and efforts of other stakeholders, such as development partners and NGOs. This support is often very welcome, but it comes with its own challenges. Unless all efforts are coordinated, considerable potential exists for duplication of activities, lack of coverage of geographical areas, and the communication of contradictory messages. Too often the left hand ends up not knowing what the right hand is doing. The Ministry of Education, Science and Sports (MoESS) has sought to prevent this from happening in Ghana by creating the School Health Education Program (SHEP), an innovative system for delivering and coordinating education-sector HIV prevention.

Description

SHEP is responsible for all school health activities in Ghana. It sets national standards for HIV prevention education in schools and coordinates the efforts of a range of nongovernment stakeholders. It aims to enable schools to increase their capacity to implement prevention education that is coherent, coordinated, and effective.

Rationale and History

SHEP was initiated by Ghana's ministries of education and health in 1992, following the government's ratification of the UN Charter on the Rights

Clara Fayorsey, consultant, conducted the interviews and collected the data for this chapter. Hilda Eghan, HIV/AIDS Secretariat; Mary Quaye, SHEP; Cynthia Bosumtwi-Sam, SHEP National Coordinator; Vincent Tay, consultant; and Albert Kpoor, consultant, provided support, encouragement, and assistance.

of the Child in 1990. SHEP is a unit within the Ghana Education Service (GES), which is part of the MoESS, the ministry responsible for pretertiary education. The program was established to integrate health education and health delivery services, to improve children's education and overall health and survival. From its inception, the program has aimed to promote the well-being of students, their families, and the community by positively influencing knowledge, attitudes, beliefs, and values about health. Throughout its history, SHEP has sought to meet its aim by training and enabling local school health coordinators and students in a range of school health issues, such as environmental health and sanitation, family life education, and food and nutrition.

As time went on, SHEP expanded its activities to integrate education-sector HIV prevention alongside its more traditional school health role. The program views the two activities as complementary, regarding good health as essential to a good education and a good education as essential to the prevention of HIV infection. With this in mind, SHEP strongly promotes the improvement of all aspects of children's health as an important means of improving school enrollment and retention. The government sees investment in children's health as a means of investing in the quality of their education and a long-term and effective means of helping them remain free of HIV.

Two principal external bodies, the Ghana AIDS Commission (GAC) and the MoESS HIV/AIDS Secretariat, have guided the unit's work in HIV prevention. GAC was set up in line with the government's policy of slowing and eventually halting the spread of AIDS by preventing new HIV infections. It aims to expand its efforts to deal in the following areas:

- Policy, advocacy, and establishment of an enabling environment

- Coordination and management of a decentralized response

- Mitigation of the economic, sociocultural, and legal impacts of HIV/AIDS

- Prevention and behavior change communication

- Treatment, care, and support

- Research, surveillance, monitoring, and evaluation

- Resource mobilization and funding arrangements.

The HIV/AIDS Secretariat was established to coordinate all HIV/AIDS interventions across agencies within MoESS.

Under the guidance of these two bodies, SHEP is mandated to implement school health activities, including HIV/AIDS education, in schools across the country. To ensure that all schools benefit from these activities, it works in collaboration with various stakeholders, including relevant governmental organizations, NGOs, community-based organizations (CBOs), faith-based organizations (FBOs), and other development partners.

The cooperation of such stakeholders—with all their energy, resources, creativity, and activity—is highly advantageous. Their presence enhances capacity, enabling many more schools and students to be reached than would be possible through government action alone. At the same time, the operation of so many different actors poses the threat that interventions delivered can be fragmented, uncoordinated, and, in the worst case, contradictory. To prevent this from happening, SHEP coordinates the activities of different partners to provide clear and common direction for their work in schools.

Aims, Objectives, and Strategies

The aim of SHEP is to facilitate the creation of well-informed and healthy students equipped with life skills that enable them to maintain healthy behaviors. The program objectives are to:

- provide skills-based health education to students

- provide students, teachers, and the school community with knowledge and skills to make informed choices for healthy behaviors

- improve the physical, social, and mental health and development of school-age children

- promote a healthy and friendly learning environment, to enhance school retention and academic competence.

The program seeks to achieve these objectives through the following strategies:

- Delivery of HIV prevention education in schools by a range of stakeholders

- Delivery of a range of additional school health interventions, including interventions on environmental health and sanitation, personal hygiene, physical education, adolescent reproductive health, safety and security, family life, drug and substance abuse, food and nutrition, and school health services

- Coordination of delivery through the use of consistent messages and a common model of implementation.

Target Groups

SHEP operates in public primary and secondary schools. Its primary target is school-going children 4–14 and their teachers. The secondary target group includes parents and school communities.

Components

SHEP does not seek to be the primary provider of training and delivery of services but rather to enable the coordination of such activity by a range of stakeholders. Its work includes the following components:

- Establishment of national guidelines to ensure consistent implementation of school-based education on HIV prevention

- Regional and district coordination of stakeholders in the content and delivery of school-based HIV prevention activities

- Sensitization of parents and members of the school community about program activities

- Capacity building of various actors to ensure maximum efficiency

- Close collaboration of SHEP coordinators with Ministry of Health counterparts at all levels.

SHEP has sought to ensure consistent implementation of school-based HIV prevention education through the development and use of a framework for delivery called the Alert model. The aim of the model is to achieve and sustain positive behavior development and change to reduce the spread of HIV among teachers, students, and the school community.

The objectives of the model are to:

- build capacity within GES to implement and sustain interventions in schools for positive behavior development and change among students, teachers, and the school community

- institutionalize mechanisms for providing schools with the tools to become HIV alert

- ensure that every school in Ghana is HIV alert

- build systems and develop the tools for assessing progress

- kick-start a campaign for national coverage of HIV prevention interventions in all primary and secondary schools.

The Alert model is built on three pillars: the teacher-led pillar, the child-led pillar, and the school community–directed pillar. Each of these pillars is described below.

Teacher-led pillar

Teachers use the integrated HIV/AIDS curricula and materials developed by GES. In addition to structured lessons, teachers use participatory methods to interact and communicate with students about HIV/AIDS (box 4.1). Methods include:

- drama and role play

- music and dance

- health talks, demonstrations, and story telling

- field trips

- films

- peer education and child-to-child activities

- health quizzes and debates

- celebration of school health days/weeks

- display of information, education, and communication materials.

Child-led pillar

Peer educators lead activities that promote positive behavior development and change using participatory child-led learning methodologies. Peer education takes place during weekly after-school sessions (sometimes called HIV/AIDS clubs) attended by groups of 14–16 students over a four-week period. Sessions are organized as discussions. Peer educators use a manual and education materials to facilitate meetings.

Box 4.1: Example of Participatory Exercise Used in Ghana

Aim: To enable students to grasp the economic impact of HIV on families, communities, and the nation as part of a social studies lesson.

Exercise: The teacher introduces a case study about the impact of HIV on a married couple and their three children. The father is unfaithful to his wife and becomes infected with HIV. He frequently falls sick and is unable to go to work.

Students are asked to discuss the economic implications of his illness for his children, his wife, his extended family, the community, and the country. As students voice their views, the teacher writes them on the blackboard and encourages students to discuss them. He or she then sums up the discussion and emphasizes the negative impact of the disease on Ghana's human resources.

Source: SHEP program manager.

Peer educators also help organize special events, including sporting events, debates, quizzes, drama, role-plays, video shows, interactions with people living with HIV/AIDS, and related activities. These activities include children from different classes and schools. Peer educators are also expected to support the activities of teachers, by making sure posters are displayed at all vantage points within the school, for example.

School community–directed pillar

Community members receive training to protect themselves against HIV and to reinforce school-based education in the home. The participation of parents is considered very important to the success of the program.

Implementation

Implementation of SHEP requires coordination at many levels (figure 4.1).

Management

The HIV/AIDS Secretariat coordinates HIV/AIDS activities within the education sector. The sector HIV/AIDS response plan is an integral part of the Education Strategic Plan for 2003–15 and the Education Sector Operational Plan 2006–08.

SHEP is situated within GES, the agency responsible for educating children aged 4–14 in kindergarten, primary school, and junior-secondary school. The program operates through a well-structured system that extends to all levels of administration (national, regional, district, and school).

Training and Support

Training and support are provided to teachers, peer educators, and school community members.

Training of teachers

Capacity building of teachers working as SHEP educators falls within the first (teacher-led) Alert pillar. This pillar contains both preservice and in-service components. MoESS plans to integrate the Alert model into the programs of teacher training colleges. In-service training takes place at the school level and is carried out by SHEP district coordinators, school health coordinators, and staff of local partners.

Figure 4.1: National, Regional, District, and School-Level Coordination of SHEP

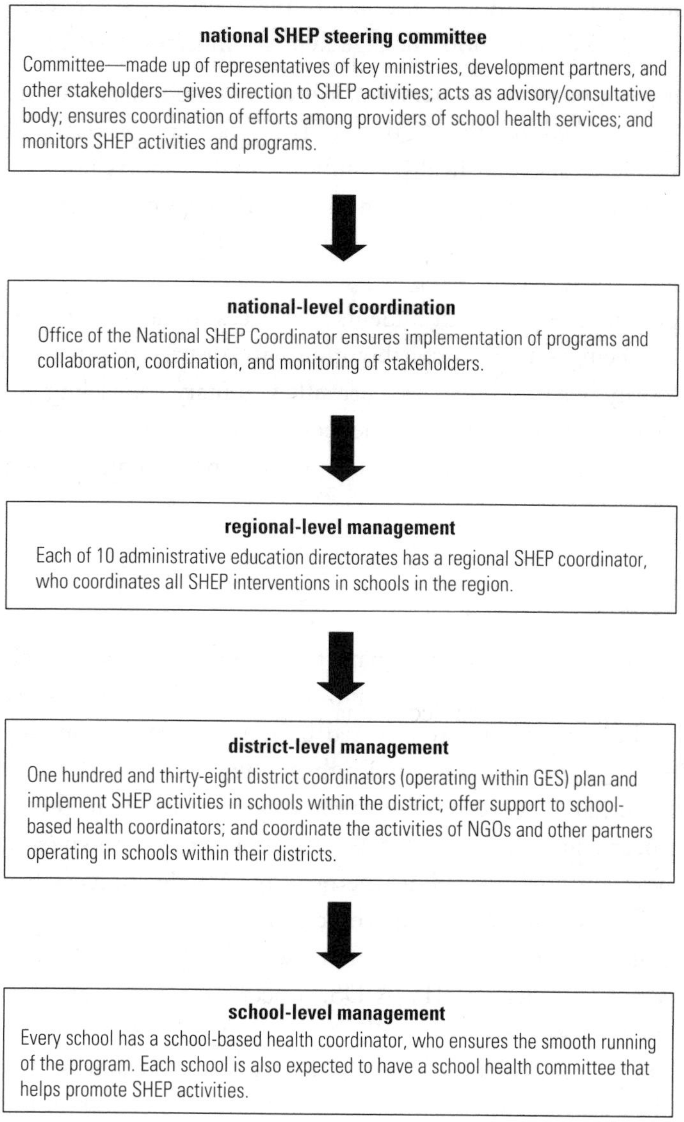

national SHEP steering committee
Committee—made up of representatives of key ministries, development partners, and other stakeholders—gives direction to SHEP activities; acts as advisory/consultative body; ensures coordination of efforts among providers of school health services; and monitors SHEP activities and programs.

national-level coordination
Office of the National SHEP Coordinator ensures implementation of programs and collaboration, coordination, and monitoring of stakeholders.

regional-level management
Each of 10 administrative education directorates has a regional SHEP coordinator, who coordinates all SHEP interventions in schools in the region.

district-level management
One hundred and thirty-eight district coordinators (operating within GES) plan and implement SHEP activities in schools within the district; offer support to school-based health coordinators; and coordinate the activities of NGOs and other partners operating in schools within their districts.

school-level management
Every school has a school-based health coordinator, who ensures the smooth running of the program. Each school is also expected to have a school health committee that helps promote SHEP activities.

Source: Authors.

In addition to developing competence on the integrated HIV/AIDS curricula, all teachers are trained in the following areas:

- Peer education

- Monitoring and evaluation

- Basic counseling skills and psychosocial support services in school (at least one male and one female teacher from each school are trained in these skills)

- Provision of HIV/AIDS education to nonteaching staff

- Planning and facilitation of training of members of parent-teacher associations (PTAs) and school management committees (SMCs).

Ongoing support for teachers is provided by school health coordinators, who are supported by the district SHEP coordinator. Each school is expected to have a school health committee that supports implementation of SHEP–related activities, including HIV/AIDS education. As part of the Alert program, teachers are required to attend at least one refresher course on HIV/AIDS every two years.

To ensure that teachers and students have access to health services, referral systems are being set up in collaboration with district health management teams. Priority health services are currently voluntary counseling and testing and treatment of STIs (national guidelines on voluntary counseling and treatment indicate that a child who is under 18 requires parental consent before accessing the service).

Selection and training of peer educators

Each school is required to nominate four children from each class from upper-primary classes to grade 3 of junior-secondary school to serve as peer educators. Peer educators are selected by their classmates on the basis of their ability to communicate in English, their motivation to work as a peer educator, and the recommendation of young people in the school. In selecting peer educators, schools take into consideration the need for a balance of boys and girls as well as the need to include students from social classes, religious affiliations, and ethnic groups.

Peer educators are trained to initiate activities that involve all children and educate each other on HIV/AIDS. A peer education manual is used to train peer educators.

GES organizes national training for a core team of trainers of peer educators. These trainers are drawn largely from the NGO community, which has experience in peer education and other participatory learning methodologies. The aim is to train trainers of peer educators and teachers together as much as possible, to harmonize and facilitate mutual reinforcement of the teacher-led and child-led pillars.

Training of school community members

The Alert model supports linkages between schools and PTAs/SMCs. Teacher trainers are responsible for training school community members. Training takes place at the district level and aims to equip PTA/SMC representatives to integrate HIV prevention into their meetings. Where PTA/SMC members have relevant skills, they are also invited to facilitate the training. At the school level, teachers who have received training in HIV prevention support the school community in planning and facilitating events that encourage positive behavior development and change in community attitudes.

Materials

Various manuals and guidelines have been developed to guide education of the various target groups of the SHEP program. GES has produced an HIV/AIDS teaching manual that includes the following:

- Information about the curriculum

- Information about participatory methods for teaching about HIV/AIDS

- Development of assertiveness skills

- Sample lesson plans showing how HIV/AIDS can be infused into general curriculum topics, such as religious and moral education, English, environmental studies, science, and Ghanaian language and culture at the preschool, primary, and junior-secondary levels.

In addition to the teachers' manual, the program has produced a peer educator's manual and a school community training manual. Other key documents include the following:

- HIV/AIDS Alert School Model Implementation Guidelines

- HIV/AIDS Manual for Basic Schools

- HIV/AIDS Manual for Secondary Schools

- HIV/AIDS Games

- School Sanitation and Hygiene Education Manual

- School Mental Health and Substance Abuse Manual

These materials are supported by a range of posters, leaflets, and booklets.

Curricular Approach, Time Allocation, and Assessment

Teaching about HIV/AIDS has been infused into the school curriculum at all school levels in a range of carrier subjects, including environmental studies, integrated science, life skills, and agricultural science. Education is delivered by a range of actors: teachers, peer educators, resource people, and NGOs.

GES has produced an HIV/AIDS curriculum that covers the following topics:

- Information on HIV/AIDS

- Information on HIV/AIDS for teachers

- Signs and symptoms

- Prevention of HIV

- Understanding and respecting people living with HIV/AIDS

- Caring for people living with HIV/ADIS

- Social and economic impact of HIV/AIDS

- Counseling.

Monitoring and Recognition

Monitoring of SHEP activities occurs at various levels and takes a variety of forms:

- The office of the national SHEP coordinator receives reports from both the regional and district levels. These reports give details of activities carried out and their impact. National-level personnel also monitor activities. Within MoESS the outcomes of all SHEP activities are presented at annual review meetings, where inputs from SHEP partners are presented. Partners are encouraged to integrate monitoring and evaluation into programs their organizations sponsor.

- Regional SHEP coordinators monitor SHEP activities within their regions by visiting program sites to ensure that standards and quality are maintained.

- SHEP coordinators and other partners involved in SHEP activities conduct monitoring at the district level. District SHEP coordinators monitor all school health implementation within the district. They are supported actively by circuit supervisors, who oversee 20 or more basic schools within each district.

- Head teachers are expected to evaluate the content and scope of teachers' lesson plans and notes to ensure that lessons integrate learning about HIV/AIDS and other aspects of school health.

A simple monitoring tool has been developed to enable district SHEP coordinators to assess the performance of the Alert model in districts or schools (table 4.1).

Table 4.1: Questions Asked to Monitor Progress toward Implementing Each Pillar of the Alert Model

TEACHER-LED PILLAR	STUDENT-LED PILLAR	SCHOOL COMMUNITY–DIRECTED PILLAR
1. What proportion of teachers was trained in the integrated HIV/AIDS curriculum?	1. How many children are enrolled in the school?	1. Has the school provided formal orientation for all PTA and SMC members on the Alert model?
2. What proportion of staff trained during last two academic years?	2. How many children have been trained and are currently working as peer educators?	2. Has the school provided formal training on HIV/AIDS for leaders of PTAs and SMCs?
3. Do teachers have access to a counselor trained in HIV/AIDS? How many trained counselors are there at this school?	3. Does every class have at least one male and one female peer educator?	3. During the past academic year, at how many PTA and school management committee meetings was HIV/AIDS discussed?
4. How many teachers received counseling on HIV/AIDS during the past 12 months?	4. How many active HIV/AIDS clubs operate in the school?	
5. Do teachers have easy access to STI treatment services in a health facility?	5. How many students belong to each of these clubs?	
6. How many teachers were able to cover all lessons and activities on HIV/AIDS planned last term?	6. On average how many students did each peer educator reach in the last academic term?	
7. How many teachers have the complete set of recommended manuals and teaching materials on HIV/AIDS?	7. How many children received at least five different lessons on HIV/AIDS in class during the last academic year?	
	8. How many children have access to educational materials on HIV/AIDS such as handouts, brochures, and pamphlets?	
	9. How many trained counselors serve children in this school (including children themselves)?	
	10. How many children received counseling services from these sources during the past academic year?	
	11. Does a functional STI referral system reach children in this school?	
	12. If so, how many STI cases were identified during the past 12 months in this school?	

Source: Alert Handbook.

An important aspect of the Alert model is its certification and award system. Based on their progress in implementing the model (as measured using the monitoring tool), schools are identified as being in one of three phases:

- Inception phase: School has finalized preparations to work toward full implementation of the Alert model.

- Pass phase: Implementation of the process is under way.

- Alert phase: Alert model is fully implemented in a satisfactory manner.

Schools in different phases are awarded color-coded flags to be flown alongside the national flag, color-coded ribbons for students, certificates, and citations. Additional recognition for achievement is given through the award of plaques and prizes, publicity in the media, travel opportunities to HIV conferences, workshops and activities, best teacher award schemes, and visits by celebrities.

Partnerships and Funding

SHEP works in active partnership with a large number of NGOs and civil society organizations (CSOs) —including Child and Teen Focus, Plan Ghana, Prolink, the National Partnership for Children's Trust, Save Foundation International, World Education, and Youth Horizons—to implement school-based HIV/AIDS and health interventions. Some organizations are active in many different districts and large numbers of schools. Others work on a much smaller scale.

These interventions have focused largely on awareness creation and behavior change activities using teaching-learning approaches such as peer education and edutainment (drama, video shows, story telling, and folklore) (box 4.2). They have developed a variety of materials for school children.

As a result of use of the Alert model, the activities of partners now take place in a much more coordinated manner. Interventions are coordinated by a single unit (GES/SHEP) and synchronized with the Annual Education Sector Operational Plan, enabling common standards of delivery, content, and quality to be met.

SHEP receives funding from the government and from a range of donors, including the Danish International Development Agency (DANIDA), the Department for International Development (DFID), the Japan International Cooperation Agency (JICA), the United Nations Children's Fund (UNICEF), the U.S. Agency for International Development (USAID), and the World Health Organization (WHO). The multiplicity of donor activities in the implementation framework makes it difficult to estimate program costs.

Coordination of Stakeholders

Regional and district SHEP coordinators work with local stakeholders to coordinate the implementation of HIV prevention education in their areas. Coordinators discuss with stakeholders the aims, objectives, and activities they wish to implement in local schools. Close attention is paid to ensuring

---

Box 4.2: Examples of NGO Programs Operating in Ghana: World Education and Child and Teen Focus

---

World Education established the Strengthening HIV/AIDS Partnership in Education (SHAPE) program in Ghana in 2001. In its first phase, the program worked in about 90 schools and communities in 15 districts. In 2005 the program entered a second phase, which aims to:

- improve the knowledge, attitudes, and behaviors of students, parents, and teachers regarding HIV/AIDS
- increase the number of school-based activities related to HIV education, prevention, and support
- increase the capacity of the education sector to respond to the epidemic
- increase the capacity of teacher training colleges to address HIV/AIDS.

SHEP staff have worked with SHAPE in a variety of areas, including:

- policy development
- preservice and in-service teacher training in participatory methodologies
- school-based risk-reduction education
- participatory and peer-to-peer education (life skills for students and teachers)
- involvement of people living with HIV/AIDS (providing unique perspectives and experiences that can help young people reduce their own risk and eliminate bias toward people living with HIV/AIDS)
- better linkages with health services (particularly youth-friendly services)
- strengthened systems of nonformal and community education, particularly for out-of-school youth.

Partnership is a reciprocal relationship. As well as providing input into design and implementation of SHAPE activities, SHEP staff have also received capacity-building training and expert input from SHAPE. CSOs deliver many SHAPE activities on the ground. District SHEP coordinators oversee implementation of such interventions.

Child and Teen Focus is a small-scale NGO that aims to reach adolescents with information on sexuality and to provide counseling services on adolescent reproductive health. The program operates in the Ga West District of the Greater Accra Region of Ghana. A partner of World Education's SHAPE program, it undertakes teacher training; training of peer educators (in schools and communities); counseling services to schools and communities; radio programs; interactive lectures; and workshops and seminars.

SHEP district coordinators play an important role in enabling Child and Teen staff to collaborate and interact with schools in their area. They also help heads of schools select teaching staff for program training.

---

that proposed activities are in line with the General Education Services HIV/AIDS Education Curriculum and Teachers' Manual and the Alert model. Should stakeholders deviate significantly from the content or operation of the activities agreed with the SHEP coordinator, permission to operate within schools may be withdrawn. In support of stakeholders,

SHEP coordinators attend stakeholder trainings to offer their support, guidance, and advice to trainers and trainees.

Advocacy

SHEP uses a number of advocacy strategies to encourage enhanced participation and support of program aims and activities by students, implementers, policy makers, and decision makers. Strategies include the following:

- Sensitization/creation of awareness

- Collaboration, networking, and partnership

- Capacity building

- Human resource development

- Operational research

- Development and review of information, education, and communication materials

- Distribution of circulars

- Feedback to decision makers.

Lessons Learned

The program has not yet been evaluated. Nevertheless, several lessons have been learned.

Ensuring Consistency

SHEP and the Alert model provide a strong basis for delivering uniform, high-quality HIV prevention education across Ghana. The system that has been developed allows all stakeholders to operate within clear and transparent boundaries toward a common effort. Bringing together so many different partners with so many different needs and priorities is not without its complications, however. Ensuring and maintaining standards remains a challenge.

The efficient operation of SHEP district coordinators has been found to be vital to ensuring consistency of approach. Coordinators work with partners to shape proposals for work in schools to ensure that they fit within the established model and guidelines. Coordinator participation in stakeholder training is also key for ensuring consistency.

When consistency is not maintained (that is, stakeholders deviate significantly from the national model), it is essential that coordinators carefully document the issues. This documentation is then used to put activities back on track by ensuring that partners follow guidelines. Failing this, permission to provide education on HIV/AIDS is withdrawn.

Ensuring Motivation

At about 3 percent, the prevalence of HIV in Ghana is much lower than that of many other countries in Africa—and sentinel survey evidence suggests that prevalence may be declining. Where prevalence is perceived to be low, it can be difficult to maintain motivation, even when a problem continues to represent a major public health issue.

A key aspect of the Alert model has been the idea of its becoming a recognizable "brand" within the education sector. The model's award levels and associated benefits are intended to maintain schools' motivation for activities. It is hoped that schools in the area will feel the competitive urge to match or outperform the successes of their peers.

Increasing the Level and Stability of Resources

The role of SHEP district coordinators is essential to making SHEP and the Alert model work. But because coordinators are not linked to specific programs, they are often underresourced. The lack of funding hampers coordinators' ability to travel to schools to perform their duties.

SHEP has sought greater financial stability and resources for its coordinators by incorporating SHEP activities into district budgets. The situation could also be improved by providing SHEP with a clear budget line in the overall government budget.

Conclusion

SHEP coordinates the efforts, actions, and resources of a range of stakeholders to enable an education sector response to HIV that reaches as many of Ghana's schools as possible. Its structure enables implementation, collaboration, and coordination at all levels of government.

Annex 4.1

SHEP Attainment of Impact Benchmarks

BENCHMARK	ATTAINMENT/COMMENTS
1. Identifies and focuses on specific sexual health goals	Partial. Curriculum seeks to educate students broadly about HIV/AIDS, its transmission, and impact.
2. Focuses narrowly on specific behaviors that lead to sexual health goals	No. HIV prevention is integrated within a range of school health messages.
3. Identifies and focuses on sexual psychosocial risk and protective factors that are highly related to each of these behaviors	No.
4. Implements multiple activities to change each of the selected risk and protective factors	✓
5. Actively involves youth by creating a safe social environment	✓ Peer educators have been trained. Clubs have been formed in schools across the country.
6. Employs a variety of teaching methods designed to involve participants and have them personalize the information	✓
7. Conveys clear message about sexual activity and condom or contraceptive use and continually reinforces that message	Partial. National messages on sexual behavior and condom use are conveyed, but focus in schools is on abstinence.
8. Includes effective curricula and activities appropriate to the age, sexual experience, and culture of participating students	✓ Curricula are designed to be age appropriate.
9. Increases knowledge by providing basic, accurate information about the risks of teen sexual activity and methods of avoiding intercourse or using protection against pregnancy and STIs	✓
10. Uses some of the same strategies to change perceptions of peer values, to recognize peer pressure to have sex, and to address that pressure	✓ Peer education is an important aspect of the Alert model's child-led pillar.
11. Identifies specific situations that might lead to sex, unwanted sex, or unprotected sex and identifies methods of avoiding those situations or getting out of them	✓ Use of scenario building and role-play is encouraged.
12. Provides modeling of and practice with communication, negotiation, and refusal skills to improve both skills and self-efficacy in using those skills	✓ Communication skills are important aspect of curricula.

Source: Authors.

Annex 4.2

Contact Information

National Coordinator
School Health Education Program (SHEP)
Ghana Education Service
Accra, Ghana
Tel./fax: +233-21-244229
SHEP materials may be obtained by contacting the national SHEP coordinator.

The Jerusalem AIDS Project at a Glance

Number of schools participating: About 40–70 primary and secondary schools a year. Contact with more than 500 schools is maintained through Internet availability of program materials, a Web chat site, and a telephone hotline.

Coverage: Nationwide; 30,000 learners were reached in 2004. Since the initiation of the program, more than 500,000 learners have been reached in Israel. The model has also been used in 27 other countries.

Target groups: Youth 13–21 in schools and informal educational settings; secondary target audience includes men and women in uniform, teachers, and parents.

Components: Program provides AIDS education in and out of schools, AIDS education to the uniformed services, a telephone hotline, outreach to parents and the community, and training of teachers and others.

Establishment and duration: Begun in 1986; envisaged as a long-term, permanent program

Management: Jerusalem AIDS Project, an NGO staffed entirely by volunteers

Role of Ministry of Education: Provides partial funding; since 2005 collaborates in diffusion of Internet-based program in schools

Costs: About $1.75 per learner in 2004

Key evaluation results: Program increased knowledge about HIV/AIDS, reduced negative attitudes toward people living with HIV/AIDS, increased tolerance of homosexuality, raised condom use slightly among sexually active students, and increased discussion between parents and children of issues related to HIV.

The Jerusalem AIDS Project, Israel

> We want to increase the knowledge about HIV/AIDS, its causes, its prevention. We want to decrease fear of AIDS. We want to provide tools for coping with HIV/AIDS cases in schools. We want to increase knowledge about the human immune system. We want to promote responsible decisions about one's health.
>
> *JAIP Program Manager*

Since its creation in 1986, Israel's Jerusalem AIDS Project (JAIP) has acquired extensive experience in responding to the challenge of providing a long-term, sustainable, and scaled-up response to HIV/AIDS.[1] The project's volunteers have provided regular HIV/AIDS education to thousands of young Israelis, both in and outside of schools.

The program has responded to the changing understanding of HIV and the evolution, both in Israel and globally, from fear to complacency. Its approach has proved successful both in Israel and in the 27 other countries that have adopted its materials and approach.

Description

JAIP is a volunteer-based nongovernmental organization (NGO), based in Jerusalem, that, upon request, implements HIV/AIDS education activities in primary and secondary schools and among members of the police and armed forces. Most of the program's financial support comes from grants and donations. It school-based education activities are partly financed by the Ministry

Silvia Jonas, consultant, conducted the interviews and collected the data for this chapter. Hanni Oren, JAIP chair, and Inon Schenker, senior HIV/AIDS prevention specialist, provided support, encouragement, and assistance.

of Education. The Ministry of Health provides JAIP with funding for a telephone hotline, which provides information and advice about HIV/AIDS.

Rationale and History

JAIP aims to prevent HIV infection, increase awareness of HIV/AIDS, encourage changes in attitudes and behavior, and increase acceptance of people living with HIV/AIDS. Through the work of its volunteer educators, it seeks to facilitate communication about HIV through a triangular model that involves students, parents (and the community at large), and school staff (figure 5.1).

The program began in 1986, as schools in Jerusalem began to request basic factual information about HIV/AIDS. Early lesson plans were developed by Inon Schenker, an HIV prevention specialist. The successful use of these materials in a small number of schools led other schools to request them. Such demand led to the creation of an expert group that developed the concepts, methods, and content of a systematic program for use in schools in Israel and elsewhere. The program that was developed is run by JAIP, an NGO that works closely with Israel's schools.

Israel's context presents the program with particular opportunities and challenges. The incidence of HIV in the country is low. When the program started, there was fear that Israel would experience an epidemic affecting many thousands of people. As time has gone by, this has not occurred, creating some complacency about the risks of infection. Yet with immigration from highly affected regions (including Eastern Europe and Ethiopia), the potential for increased transmission is ever present. At the

Figure 5.1: The JAIP Triangular Model

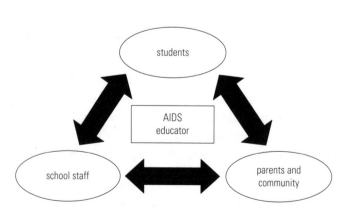

Source: JAIP.

same time, Israel's high school enrollment rates for both boys and girls and strong cultural emphasis on education and literacy lend considerable support to the program's work.

> The whole topic of HIV/AIDS is not a taboo anymore. People are not ashamed to talk about it. However, they have become indifferent, which is not better.
>
> *JAIP Implementer*

Early in the life of the program, positive evaluations and reports by academic and international agencies led to requests to adapt the approach for use in other countries. Doing so has enabled insights from different cultures and contexts to be shared, enriching the application of the approach all over the world. Argentina, Brazil, Costa Rica, the Dominican Republic, Ecuador, El Salvador, Germany, Guatemala, Honduras, Jordan, Nepal, Panama, Kazakhstan, the Kyrgyz Republic, Lithuania, Peru, the Philippines, the Russian Federation, Rwanda, Uganda, the United States, Venezuela, the West Bank and Gaza, and Yugoslavia have all adopted the JAIP model for use in their national curricula or conducted training for teachers and other AIDS educators on how to tailor the approach for use in their schools.

Aims, Objectives, and Strategies

The principal aim of the program is to save the lives of young people by preventing them from being infected with HIV. The program also aims to promote acceptance of people living with HIV/AIDS, to decrease fear of AIDS, and to promote greater openness about discussing the disease. An overarching goal is to enhance health promotion attitudes and activities in young people by promoting communication about HIV/AIDS among students, their parents/community, and school staff.

The objectives of the program are to:

- provide clear information about HIV/AIDS and the human immune system to all members of the community

- enable young people to acquire skills and strategies that will help them avoid infection

- provide tools for coping with HIV/AIDS cases in schools

- enable young people to take responsible decisions about their health

- position HIV prevention within school health promotion.

The program seeks to meet its objectives through a range of strategies, including the following:

- Delivering AIDS education in schools through volunteer AIDS educators

- Working with communities and parents to create supportive environments for education

- Supporting community action for health change through World AIDS Day activities

- Increasing knowledge and understanding of the sexual attitudes and behavior of young people through research on 15- to 18-year-olds

- Disseminating research findings on the sexual attitudes and behavior of young people to policy makers and other stakeholders, with the objective of enhancing policy development

- Increasing the capacity of other NGOs to deal with HIV/AIDS and sexual health issues by offering training workshops.

Target Groups

The primary target population is primary- and secondary-school students. The program reaches 40–70 schools and about 30,000 students a year.

Secondary target groups include teachers, parents, and the wider community and members of the police and armed forces, especially those undertaking national service. The program reaches 150,000–200,000 parents, men and women in uniform, school staff, and community leaders each year.

Approaches

The key setting for conducting education on HIV prevention is the school. Outreach to parents and community complements school-based education. Parents are encouraged to discuss HIV/AIDS with their children through "coffee and AIDS afternoons."

The program aims to help young people make their own decisions, based on sound information delivered by (slightly older) peer AIDS educators. The program also works with religious organizations, communities, parents, policy makers, and NGO staff.

JAIP education on HIV/AIDS and sexuality takes place in an open and positive manner. Sexuality is depicted as something natural; educators strive to create an atmosphere in which students feel comfortable talking about sex and sexually transmitted diseases (STDs). Learners are encouraged to share their experiences and ask questions throughout the sessions. By allowing learners to ask questions and share their views, educators get a feel for their learning needs.

> I speak with my classes in an open way and I give them [the learners] the feeling they can ask every question they want.
> They [the students] are encouraged to talk about their own experiences in a dialogue. This way, we create dynamic lessons like a ping-pong game.
>
> *JAIP Implementers*

Another important aspect of JAIP is the humanizing of HIV/AIDS, which is done by inviting people living with HIV/AIDS to talk with learners about their experiences. Program implementers have found that meeting with people with the disease also increases learners' acceptance of and respect for them.

> They hear my personal story of how I got infected and how I live with it now. To see a person infected by HIV, who is close to them by age is enough to make them respect individuals' rights and decrease stigma.
>
> *JAIP Implementer*

The program also promotes (but does not provide) HIV testing. It provides information about where learners can get condoms and how to use them. It operates a free HIV/AIDS hotline, which provides information and counseling. Following a successful pilot, the hotline service was extended to the Internet in 2006. Young people, who are very active users of the Internet in Israel, can use it for live chats with hotline counselors.

> We teach then to raise the issue of STIs with their partners; we teach them to insist on safe sex; we teach them to have open and honest talks with partners before having sex.
>
> *JAIP Implementer*

The program uses a wide variety of methods to deliver its messages. These include group discussions, lectures, printed materials, videos, dramas, songs, games, and cartoons.

Components

The JAIP program includes six components:

- AIDS education in schools

- AIDS education out of school

- AIDS education to men and women in uniform

- Telephone hotline

- Outreach to parents and the community

- Training of teachers and others

  Each of these components is discussed in the next section.

Implementation

Management

JAIP is a volunteer-based, national and international NGO. It has an active board, which includes professionals from various disciplines and people living with HIV/AIDS.

The program manager is responsible for the day-to-day running of the organization. An important part of this work involves ensuring effective coordination between schools and AIDS educators. Such coordination relieves educators of having to make arrangements with the schools in which they work.

Methodology

The main approach is interactive and participative classroom teaching delivered by JAIP volunteers. The program provides some AIDS education after school, through clubs run by youth organizations. AIDS educators lead activities such as role-plays and discussions, and they show videos about HIV/AIDS. Since 2005 materials from JAIP's HIV prevention program have been posted on the Internet, enabling participation to be maintained among more than 500 schools. The program is also delivered to young people in the military, giving them a "booster shot of AIDS education" before they join their units. JAIP trains medical officers and sends an annual "Note on HIV/AIDS," signed by the army surgeon-general, to all men and women serving in the Israeli Defense Forces (IDF). On World AIDS Day JAIP, together with the IDF, publishes a poster to be displayed in every base.

The mainstay of the program is teaching about HIV/AIDS in schools. This is done through workshops organized upon request of the school or community. HIV/AIDS is said to be "mentioned in biology and science classes," but comprehensive teaching of the subject is not compulsory. Lessons are therefore not an integral part of the regular curriculum. The program's educators provide HIV education as something on its own, at a time arranged by the school.

Before going into classrooms, AIDS educators deliver an introductory lecture to school staff. The lecture lasts about two hours. It aims to sensitize staff about the program and to elicit their support, educate staff about HIV/AIDS, and highlight the role of school staff in the triangular model shown in figure 5.1. After the lecture and discussion, the AIDS educator leaves materials for the school library, a plan of action and timetable for classwork, and contact numbers school staff can call with questions. Educators' visits are accompanied by an exhibition about HIV/AIDS in the schools, which remains there for about two weeks.

Classroom teaching usually takes place over four academic hours, spread over two days. On the first day, students fill out a short KAP (knowledge, attitude, and practice) questionnaire. A short lecture is then given using cartoon flip charts included in the program materials pack. Students then work in pairs and small groups on questions concerning sensitive issues and decision making using participatory role-play and other methods.

AIDS educators use the educational kits (described below) provided by the program. The kits enable them to teach about HIV/AIDS in a manner that is participative, interactive, and challenging. The program is modular, allowing topics to be added or dropped depending on the needs of particular communities. Topics covered include:

- HIV/AIDS transmission and impact

- Abstinence, Being faithful, and Condom use

- Behavior change

- Behavioral and life-skills development

- HIV testing

- Communication skills

- Moral behavior and social values education

- Relationships

- Peer pressure

- Human and child rights

- Public health policy

> We received basic knowledge on the virus, the disease, prevention and testing and also on the social aspects. We also gained some communication skills and info where we could be tested.
>
> *Students*

The first day of teaching concludes with the setting of tasks to be undertaken before the next session. These include interviewing parents and members of the community, reading some texts, and retaking the KAP (so that JAIP can measure impact).

Our motto is "It is your life. You have the information – now it is up to you to decide how you want to live it."

According to my experience, the best way to [teach HIV prevention] is to give as much "dry" information as possible to start with and then to shift the lecture into an open conversation where the children do most of the talking with each other under my guidance. In these discussions all themes are tackled such as safe sex, love, sexual behavior, boys-girls issues and peer influence.

The youth do not have enough concrete information about the disease, the stigmas are more common. Therefore you have to put things correctly and then let them "stir things up" in the classroom. This way the children suddenly hear the other's opinion in this issue. Such conversations usually do not develop by themselves because of embarrassment. The program gives them a "safe place" to talk about it.

You need a lot of highly motivated volunteers, a good trainer, a good concept and the support of the government. In the classroom itself you have to be patient, you have to be sensitive and you have to be able to adopt the language of the kids from today. Otherwise they will not listen to you.

JAIP Implementers

I believe that half a class is better than a whole one. A small number of students provides an intimate atmosphere and makes the children less shy and more willing to ask their questions.

JAIP Implementer

Being taught about AIDS was a little embarrassing at first. But afterwards we did small groups, which was good.

Students

Several days after the first lesson, a second session occurs, emphasizing skill building. It uses debates (for example, should students or teachers with HIV be allowed to attend school?); role-plays (on negotiation skills, for example); and discussions of key issues in decision making. In sessions with older learners, educators also demonstrate correct condom use. At the end of the session, students receive some written materials and the number of JAIP's telephone hotline.

Young boys face the pressure to go to prostitutes and not to use a condom. By doing this, they want to show that "they are men." There is also a lot of pressure to get tattoos or piercings. We tackle the problem through explanation and discussions.

JAIP Manager

Another very important component of the program for secondary-school students is the inclusion of a visit by a young person living with HIV. This session occurs at the end or beginning of the program in a particular school and lasts for about 1–1 1/2 hours. It addresses questions of stigma and discrimination. It is very important in changing attitudes.

> The most effective approach we have is the personal meeting with an HIV infected person. She comes with us to the lectures and tells the children the story about how she got infected, It is very emotional and thus, for sure, the children will remember it.
>
> I am HIV infected. I tell my personal story, how I got the disease, which mistakes I made and how I live with it now. I try to show the kids how important it is to have the self-confidence to insist on using a condom.
>
> *JAIP Implementers*

The structure of the program means that most young Israelis will be exposed to activities four or five times as they grow up: once in primary school, two or three times in secondary school, and once during military service.

Telephone Hotline

Trained counselors associated with the program operate a telephone hotline that can be called by young people concerned about HIV/AIDS.

Training

About 4,000 JAIP volunteers have been trained in Israel. A similar number has been trained in the other countries in which the program operates. JAIP also trains new teachers, school nurses, and staffs of other NGOs.

> Once a year the program advertises for second- or third-year medical students who wish to become volunteer AIDS educators. School teachers don't show enthusiasm to talk on the issue. Explaining is hard for them. That is why we like the medical students and other volunteers.

Interested students submit an application form with a copy of their C.V. A selection committee reviews the applications and chooses candidates with experience working with youth and evidence of the motivation and ability to volunteer for at least one year.

At its inception the program trained some high school students to be peer educators, but it did not find them as effective as medical students. According to one program implementer, "The children do not take it as seriously as they would do if there were an adult teaching them, and sometimes the peer educators delivered wrong information." Biology teachers were also trained to teach the curriculum but were found not to be as effective as volunteers.

Volunteers undergo a five-day course of training in all aspects of the program approach and program materials. Training occurs through plenary lectures and small-group exercises that cover the following topics:

- Risk taking (sex, drugs, and alcohol)

- HIV/AIDS basics

- Gender issues

- Pregnancy

- Child psychology

- Religious issues

- Communication skills

- Class facilitation skills (training also includes a meeting with a person living with HIV)

The program manager accompanies educators on their first visits to schools. Volunteers regularly receive updated materials and newsletters. The program manager meets every second month with active volunteers to supervise their work.

Hotline counselors are often university students of social work, psychology, or allied health professions. On selection, they receive a structured course of training that lasts approximately 60 hours and includes role-plays, teaching, and counseling techniques. Every two months, counselors are invited to attend a two- to three-hour refresher training session that includes updates, reviews, and supervision.

Materials

Two educational kits have been developed, one for use with primary-school students (*Explaining AIDS to Children*), another for use with secondary-school students (*The Immune System and AIDS*). The kits include a teacher's guide, cartoons, flip charts, booklets, posters, stickers, condoms, and pre- and postintervention questionnaires. Materials are regularly modified to keep them up to date and to take account of lessons learned in their use.

The cartoon approach means that the kits can be used in any country, with a diverse range of age groups. The detailed teachers' guides included in the kits have been published in Hebrew, Arabic, English, French, German, Nepalese, Portuguese, Russian, and Spanish.

> The materials are funny so we are less afraid. They are good for different ages. Like Asterix . . .
>
> *Student*

Other material, including journal articles, Power Point slides, newspaper clippings, and materials from the Joint United Nations Progamme on HIV/AIDS (UNAIDS) and other relevant agencies, supplement the kits. Practical information about HIV testing sites, including hospitals' telephone numbers, is also provided. Educators can access additional resources from the JAIP's resource center.

Advocacy

Information about the program is published in newspapers, over the Internet, and on posters and stickers. Staff associated with the program also participate in television programs viewed by young people.

The program has lobbied the Israeli parliament to develop a national policy on HIV/AIDS and education and to include HIV/AIDS education in the school curriculum. Program staff also meet regularly with staff of the ministries of education and health, and they remain in continuous contact with the media.

Costs

In 2004 the program received funding from private and public foundations, schools, and Ministry of Education grants. The program has never had any paid staff or managers. Everyone associated with the program is a volunteer, allowing the program to run at very little cost (table 5.1).

Table 5.1: Annual Cost of JAIP Program, 2004

(U.S. dollars)

ITEM	AMOUNT
Salaries	0
Transportation	4,000
Training	25,000
Office administration	3,500
Materials development	3,000
Materials distribution	10,000
Evaluation	1,000
Advocacy	5,000
Total	51,500

Source: JAIP.

Evaluation

Routine evaluation of aspects of the program has occurred since its launch. Pre- and post-tests are used at each of the program's training workshops. Principals complete school evaluation forms after the conclusion of work in each school.

Evaluation of Program in Israel

Pretesting of the two curricula and teaching aids was conducted in 1986 using a questionnaire on students' needs for information about HIV/AIDS and possible approaches to teaching. The structured, open-ended questionnaire was completed by 26 experts in public health, education, medicine, psychology, and related fields. The responses suggested that there was an urgent need to provide accurate and balanced information on HIV/AIDS to primary-school students to reduce fears elevated by media reports. Responses also confirmed and endorsed JAIP's proposed approach, the curricula, and teaching aids. Since 1989 pre– and post–Knowledge, Attitudes, Practices, and Beliefs (KAPB) questionnaires have been administered to parents and students who attend sessions at participating schools.

In 1994 a quasi-experimental study, using anonymous questionnaires, examined the effectiveness of the program in secondary public schools (Schenker 1998). The questionnaires measured KAP changes in intervention and control groups two to four months post baseline ($N = 932$). Significant changes ($p < .001$) were found in KAP:

- Mean knowledge scores rose 5.6 points to 67.4 (standard deviation = 20.0).

- Negative attitudes toward people living with HIV/AIDS fell 0.81 points on a 1–5 scale (standard deviation = 0.76).

- Although not a stated target of the program, tolerance toward homosexuality rose 0.10 points on a 1–5 scale (standard deviation = 0.93).

- Reported lifetime condom use increased from 42.4 percent to 44.1 percent.

- The percentage of children who would talk with a parent about HIV rose from 23.1 percent to 24.1 percent.

- The intervention did not result in sexual initiation among participants who were not sexually active.

- There was no reported change in the levels of substance abuse.

Participants were very satisfied with the program (3.73 on a 1–4 scale), with 82.4 percent reporting that all schools should provide JAIP classes,

77.7 percent reporting increased awareness of HIV/AIDS, 53.6 percent reporting that the program had caused them to think afresh about their health, and 10.9 percent reporting a decrease in risk-taking behaviors. There were no statistically significant differences in the observed KAP changes among students taught by biology teachers and students taught by medical school students.

Anonymous questionnaires were used to evaluate the JAIP training of trainers model in 1995–96 (Galardo 1996). With a response rate of 60 percent (30 out of 50), overall satisfaction from the training activity was high, with 23.3 percent rating it excellent, 43.3 percent rating it very good, 23.3 percent rating it good, and 10.1 percent rating it poor. Seventy percent of respondents reported being highly motivated to introduce HIV prevention activities within the following two to three months.

Evaluation of Program in Latin America

JAIP's approach has been introduced in Asia, Europe, and Latin America, following requests from government ministries, NGOs, and interested individuals for assistance in setting up HIV prevention programs. JAIP volunteers traveled abroad to introduce the program design and provide training. Country organizers then took responsibility for the ongoing activity of the program.

An assessment of the effectiveness of JAIP's teacher training was conducted in five Latin American countries (Cost Rica, El Salvador, Guatemala, Honduras, and Peru). Responses to 1,272 questionnaires administered before and after the training revealed that teachers' mean knowledge rose 14 percentage points, from 74.39 (standard deviation = 16.6) to 88.4 (standard deviation = 11.6) (Erbstein, Greenblatt, and Schenker 1996). Attitude change was even more dramatic: before the workshop, 35 percent of participants were ready to isolate people living with HIV/AIDS from society. Following the workshop this figure dropped to just 1 percent. Before the workshop 60 percent of participants considered AIDS to be a frightening disease; this figure fell to 36 percent after the workshop. The mean satisfaction was 2.77 score on a 1–3 scale (standard deviation = 0.47).

Lessons Learned

Responding to the Changing Context of HIV/AIDS

Over the course of its operation, JAIP continually has had to respond to the evolving context of HIV/AIDS in Israel. In the early days of the program, when it was believed that HIV could be a major problem, there was overwhelming demand for the program's activities. In recent years, as HIV prevalence has declined, there has been a reduction of interest.

> People say, "AIDS is not a problem any more."
>
> *Program Manager*

The program has responded to complacency by undertaking sustained advocacy to schools and communities. Advocacy activities include providing information about the need to remain vigilant about HIV/AIDS, explaining the program to communities through formal and informal meetings and outreach to schools, and demonstrating the effectiveness of the program through recommendations of people who have experienced it.

Keeping the Program Approach Up to Date

Knowledge of HIV/AIDS has changed significantly since the inception of the program. A constant challenge has been continuously updating and improving activities in light of changing knowledge and understanding.

Throughout its history, the program has constantly sought to refine its activities to ensure that its impact is maximized. Examples of the ways in which the program has changed over time include the decision in 1995 to add a stronger dimension on human rights to the program and to develop subcomponents to meet the needs of non-Hebrew speakers, including Arab students. In 2000, program approaches were modified to take into account new approaches to treatment of and testing for HIV.

> The kit is now very old; it should be adjusted to new techniques and devices, for example by using the Internet.
>
> *JAIP Implementer*

Interacting with Religious Authorities

> The religious authorities reject the program and do not want to acknowledge HIV as a dangerous disease that can hit everyone.
>
> *JAIP Implementer*

Objections to the program from religious conservatives, particularly religious parties in the government, have presented the program with challenges.

Religious communities in Israel are almost entirely free of the disease. Hence there has been little demand for HIV education occur in such constituencies. It has been far more important to ensure that conservative interests do not block the provision of HIV education to other parts of society. Doing so has taken intense advocacy and considerable sensitivity. Program leaders consistently underline the organization's professionalism and achievements and ensure religious conservatives that it is not seeking to undermine their values. JAIP helped build confidence by training workshops for education and health sectors in the religious sector about HIV/AIDS. Condoms were not the main feature of such training, which focused instead on the scientific review of the evidence about HIV/AIDS.

In secular public schools, 10–12 percent of students come from conservative or moderately religious families. The participative approach employed by the program was found to be very valuable in ensuring that teaching was helpful to all. Emphasis on informed decision making by adolescents allowed room for the importance of family values, traditions, and religiosity to be expressed. JAIP sought to provide information and skills rather than to promote any particular response. If students felt uncomfortable participating in particular activities (such as cucumber condom-wearing exercises), they did not have to participate. They were, however, exposed to the fact that condoms are one way to help protect oneself against HIV/AIDS.

Recruiting Volunteers

The project relies on volunteers and accesses fresh inputs of energy and enthusiasm with each successive wave that joins the project. Despite Israel's strong culture of volunteering, however, finding enough volunteers to run the program is a constant challenge.

> The biggest difficulty is to keep the volunteer spirit alive enough to make people continue their work for us and to find even more volunteers to join us.
>
> It is very hard to keep on volunteering for a program like JAIP once you have a job. I think it is harder and harder to find volunteers who are willing to dedicate time for the program.
>
> *JAIP Implementers*

Medical students have a culture of volunteering. Good publicity, small scholarships, and excellent training ensure their participation. The possibility of participating in international training is another incentive.

Replicating the Program in Other Countries

Requests from other countries presented JAIP with the challenge of introducing an approach tailored to one cultural context into very different contexts. One of the main educational differences between Israel and some of the countries in which the approach has been used is Israel's high enrollment rates for both boys and girls and the strong cultural emphasis on education and literacy. It could be that some of the more formal teaching-learning methods used in the program (such as lectures) are especially well suited to learners in Israel.

JAIP officials responded quickly to requests and made clear what they could and could not deliver and when. Replication followed a single set of ground rules:

- A model or program cannot be transferred from one culture to another without proper cultural adaptation. A needs assessment is essential to identifying how the program must be adapted.

- Partnerships can be formed with a wide range of local associates, including governments and NGOs. It is essential that partners take initiative and responsibility for seeing that the approach is used in schools.

- The use of the JAIP curriculum should be approved by the national government.

- Replication must commence with effective training of teachers in the program's approaches. Good training is essential to the culturally sensitive application of the approach. Because of this, JAIP will not distribute its materials unless potential users agree to undergo training.

- Evaluation needs to be an integral part of the approach.

- JAIP does not establish an infrastructure in other countries but does provide technical support from time to time.

Replication was assisted by a number of other factors, inherent in the program's design:

- The modular design of JAIP's materials makes them easy to use in a wide range of cultures. Educators are able to tailor their teaching to the needs and sensitivities of different audiences. In conservative settings, for example, teaching can focus on abstinence. Elsewhere the approach can be on condom use.

- The fact that JAIP educators are volunteers means that they can be sent to other countries at very low cost.

- Users report that the provenance of the program in a small country like Israel meant that it tended to be received without fear that it carried any particular agenda. Its origin in a city important to many of the world's faith communities increased the likelihood that the more religious-minded would consider it legitimate and acceptable.

- The program materials are compact, simple, and robust. They can easily be carried by hand or tied to a bicycle or pack animal. Neither electricity nor audio-visual equipment is needed, making them suitable for developing-country settings.

Conclusions

One of the first school-based HIV prevention programs in the world, JAIP operates in Israel and many other countries. Its success can be related to a number of factors:

- The program has a simple, easily replicated formula that can be delivered easily to people in a wide range of contexts.

- The program's cartoon materials can be adapted to a wide range of situations.

- The program has adapted to changes in knowledge about HIV/AIDS and the cultural contexts in which the program is offered.

- The program's use of volunteer medical students as AIDS educators allows messages to be delivered by people who are both authoritative and respected and close in age and experience to learners.

- The program's contact with students over the course of their school and military careers enables messages to be repeated and reinforced in an age-appropriate fashion.

Annex 5.1

JAIP Attainment of Impact Benchmarks

BENCHMARK	ATTAINMENT/COMMENT
1. Identifies and focuses on specific sexual health goals	✓ Program is highly focused on transmission and prevention of HIV and other STIs. It seeks to enable students to take control of their own sexual lives and avoid infection.
2. Focuses narrowly on specific behaviors that lead to sexual health goals	✓ Program focuses on promotion of informed and unforced decision making about sexual relationships and seeks effective use of condoms.

(Continues on the following page)

BENCHMARK	ATTAINMENT/COMMENT
3. Identifies and focuses on sexual psychosocial risk and protective factors that are highly related to each of these behaviors	✓ Program focuses on enabling students to take control of their own sexual lives, teaching strategies such as avoiding risky places and behaviors, how to say "no," how to use condoms, and so forth.
4. Implements multiple activities to change each of the selected risk and protective factors	✓ Program reaches out to students, parents, communities, and soldiers in a wide variety of ways.
5. Actively involves youth by creating a safe social environment	✓ Use of medical students to deliver program messages creates teaching environments in which students feel safe and at ease.
6. Employs a variety of teaching methods designed to involve participants and have them personalize the information	✓ Wide variety of participatory teaching methodologies is used to teach program curriculum.
7. Conveys clear message about sexual activity and condom or contraceptive use and continually reinforces that message	✓ See benchmark 2.
8. Includes effective curricula and activities appropriate to the age, sexual experience, and culture of participating students	✓ Different materials are used for primary- and secondary-school students. The cartoon nature of the materials allows their use to be easily adapted to different groups.
9. Increases knowledge by providing basic, accurate information about the risks of teen sexual activity and methods of avoiding intercourse or using protection against pregnancy and STIs	✓ Course content concerning knowledge about HIV is strong and clear.
10. Uses some of the same strategies to change perceptions of peer values, to recognize peer pressure to have sex, and to address that pressure	✓ Addressing peer pressure is a major activity of AIDS educators.
11. Identifies specific situations that might lead to sex, unwanted sex, or unprotected sex and identifies methods of avoiding those situations or getting out of them	✓ Role-plays and drama enable students to identify situations that might lead to sex and how to avoid it.
12. Provides modeling of and practice with communication, negotiation, and refusal skills to improve both skills and self-efficacy in using those skills	✓ The life-skills content of the curriculum encourages students to learn and use communication, negotiation, and refusal skills.

Source: Authors.

Annex 5.2

Contact Information

The Jerusalem AIDS Project (JAIP)
10 Heller Street, POB 7179
Jerusalem, Israel 91072
Tel: +972-2-679-7677 Fax: +972-2-679-7737
E-mail: jaipolam@yahoo.com
Web site: http://www.israaid.org.il/member_page.asp?id=11

To obtain the Jerusalem AIDS Project educational kit and World AIDS Day materials (at cost), publications, and reports, please contact the JAIP Distribution Department, at the address indicated above.

Note

1. JAIP is the name of both the AIDS education project and the organization that implements it.

References

Erbstein, S., C. L. Greenblatt, and L. Schenker. 1996. "HIV/AIDS Knowledge, Beliefs, and Attitudes among Teachers in Latin America: Lessons from Five Countries in Implementing the ISYAP Model." In *AIDS Education: Interventions in Multi-cultural Societies*, eds. I. Schenker, G. Sabar-Friedman, and F. Sy. New York: Plenum.

Erez, A., and I. Schenker. 2002. "HIV/AIDS and Peace Building in the Middle East." *Entre Nous* 53 (December): 15–16. WHO-EURO.

Gallardo, A. 1996. *Post-Workshop Monitoring and Evaluation of the First Regional Training Workshop on HIV/AIDS Education in the Middle East*. Jerusalem AIDS Project, Jerusalem.

Schenker, I. 1988. "The Immune System Approach in Teaching AIDS to Youngsters: Two Unique Programs for Schools." In *The Global Impact of AIDS*, ed. A. Fleming, J. Mann, et al., pp. 341–46. New York: A. Liss.

———. 1998. "Sex, AIDS and Israeli Youth." Poster session presented at the 12th International Conference on AIDS, Geneva.

———. 2001. "New Challenges for School AIDS Education within an Evolving AIDS Pandemic." *Prospects* 30(3): 415–34.

———. 2003. "New Health Communicators at School: Medical Students." *Entre Nous* 56 (July): 23–25. WHO-EURO.

Schenker, I., and C. Greenblatt. 1993. "Israeli Youth and AIDS: Knowledge and Attitude Changes among High-School Students Following an AIDS Education Program." *Israel Journal of Medical Science* 29(10): 41–47.

The Primary School Action for Better Health Program at a Glance

Description: Teacher-led HIV/AIDS and behavior change education for 12- to 16-year-olds

Number of schools participating: 5,000 public upper-primary schools

Coverage: Twenty-six percent of public upper-primary schools in seven of Kenya's eight provinces (the North Eastern Province is not targeted, because the HIV prevalence rate is less than 5 percent)

Target groups: School-going children in public upper-primary schools, with emphasis on girls. Secondary target group includes teachers, parents, wider community, deans of teacher training colleges, educational officers, and health workers.

Components: Program components include integration and infusion of classroom teaching throughout the curriculum; teacher and peer training; out-of-class activities (assemblies, class teacher time, question box); co-curricular activities (school health clubs, information corners); extracurricular activities (drama, singing, dance, sports); peer support; and involvement of the wider community

Duration: Begun in one district in 1999. Operated in 2,000 schools in 2002 and 5,000 since 2004. Envisaged as long-term, permanent program.

Management: Centre for British Teachers (CfBT) in partnership with the Ministry of Education, Science and Technology (MoEST) and the Ministry of Health

Roles of key partners: CfBT is responsible for daily management of the program. MoEST coordinates development of relevant policies, conducts training sessions, and facilitates monitoring and evaluation. Ministry of Health trainers facilitate trainings sessions, and the ministry supports teaching-learning in schools.

Program costs (2004): $381 per school; $76 per adult trained; and $3.18 per student reached ($5.79 per student reached where peer supporters are also trained).

Key evaluation results: Evaluation 30 months after introduction of the program revealed the following results:

- Students began having sex at a later age.

Chapter 6

- Fewer students reported having had sex in the previous three months.

- More girls reported incidents of forced sex.

- More boys reported avoiding certain places to avoid having sex.

- More girls and boys reported that a condom should always be used when engaging in sexual intercourse.

- More girls reported condom usage during last sexual encounter.

- More girls felt they could say no to sex.

- More students believed that "no" means "no."

Primary School Action for Better Health, Kenya

> The goal of the PSABH initiative is "to bring about positive behavior changes in sexual relationships of upper-primary students . . . such that the risk of HIV/AIDS transmission will be reduced. We aim to provide accurate information on prevention, promote abstinence and delay the onset of sexual activity."
>
> *Taken from "PSABH peer supporters Training Notes" (2002)*

Two key challenges facing the education sector's response to HIV/AIDS concern scale and appropriateness of response. Many programs operate well at the level of the school, ward, or district but seem unable to expand to provide the scale response that is required. Moreover, although many programs can implement teaching about HIV/AIDS, they have little understanding about whether the education provided is meeting young peoples' needs and having an impact on preventing HIV. The Government of Kenya's Primary School Action for Better Health (PSABH) Program demonstrates how these challenges can be met.

Description

PSABH is a teacher-led HIV/AIDS and behavior change education for 12- to 16-year-olds enrolled in primary school in Kenya.[1] It is a joint program of the Ministry of Education, Science and Technology (MoEST); the Centre for British Teachers (C*f*BT);[2] the Kenya Institute

---

Wairimu Muita, lecturer at the U.S. International University and researcher at Population Communication Africa, in Nairobi, conducted the interviews and collected the data for this chapter. Janet Wildish and Mary Gichuru, of the Centre for British Teachers, Nairobi, provided support, encouragement, and assistance.

of Education (KIE); and the Ministry of Health. Responding to the challenge of scale, PSABH demonstrates how the building of effective partnerships, establishment of strong management structures, and careful training can enable a program to expand quickly and widely while retaining the highest standards of quality.

Rationale and History

The C*f*BT managed the Primary School Management (PRISM) program on behalf of MoEST for five years before work began on addressing HIV/AIDS–related issues in education. During implementation of PRISM, C*f*BT and the MoEST recognized the impact HIV/AIDS was having on the school environment, student attendance and performance, and communities in general. In light of this, C*f*BT designed an HIV/AIDS behavior change intervention within the school context based on its experience.

In partnership with MoEST and the Ministry of Health, C*f*BT piloted PSABH in 250 schools in Bondo District in 1999 (figure 6.1). After initial positive impressions, the project was expanded to more schools in Nyanza Region to test the potential impact of a large-scale, school-based HIV/AIDS education intervention on student knowledge, attitudes, and behavior. The documented success of the program led MoEST, in collaboration with the Ministry of Health, to expand the program to government schools in areas with a high prevalence of HIV/AIDS. The program currently targets some 5,000 schools.

PSABH targets the "window of hope"—young people who are not infected with HIV. It is based on the belief that prevention of HIV through sexual transmission is possible if young people are provided with the correct knowledge, skills, and support they need to modify their behavior patterns.

The program works within the education system to reach students in Kenya's 19,000 primary schools. It focuses on a whole-school approach, aiming to use all aspects of school life to promote and support positive behavior patterns.

Figure 6.1: Timeline of PSABH Implementation

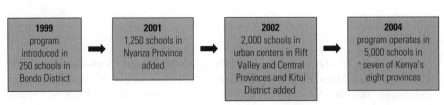

| **1999** | **2001** | **2002** | **2004** |
| program introduced in 250 schools in Bondo District | 1,250 schools in Nyanza Province added | 2,000 schools in urban centers in Rift Valley and Central Provinces and Kitui District added | program operates in 5,000 schools in seven of Kenya's eight provinces |

Source: Authors.

Aims, Objectives, and Strategies

PSABH aims to reduce the risk of HIV infection among upper-primary students by bringing about positive behavior change and providing accurate information on HIV/AIDS. The main objectives of the program are as follows:

- Improve knowledge of the transmission and prevention of HIV

- Influence students' attitudes toward sexual activity and the risk of HIV infection

- Delay the onset of sexual activity

- Enable students to control their own sexual lives and avoid infection

- Encourage young people to adopt safer sexual practices throughout their lives.

The program also seeks to improve communication about HIV/AIDS, increase compassion for people living with or affected by HIV/AIDS, help adults understand the way young people think and feel, and increase students' sense of self-worth.

The program seeks to meet its objectives through a range of strategies. These strategies include behavior and life-skills development, creation of a supportive environment for students, peer support, and the empowerment of girls.

Target Groups

Most Kenyans are able to attend primary school, while only a small minority has access to secondary education. Recognizing this, the program has maximized its use of the school system by conducting its work in upper-primary schools, where most students were (erroneously) believed not to be sexually active. The program is based in schools, because schools are believed to have a strong influence on Kenya's children and are part of a structure that enables the same interventions to be delivered throughout the country, reaching even remote areas.

The program targets students of both sexes in standards 6, 7, and 8 (ages 12–16), with an emphasis on reducing the vulnerability of girls. Supported by education and health workers, the program trains teachers and parents to deliver an integrated program of HIV/AIDS education and behavior change. The program's secondary target is adults, including education officers (at all levels), health workers, teachers, parents, and community representatives.

Approaches

Program messages are delivered through the following mechanisms:

- Group discussions of cultural and gender issues

- Drama, song, and dance

- Videos

- Lectures

- Printed materials

- Problem solving and planning.

The approach used depends on the objective. Lectures are used to provide information about HIV and other sexually transmitted infections (STIs). Interactive methodologies that involve students in planning and problem solving are used to effect behavior change.

Components

PSABH includes five components:

- Integrating and infusing teaching about HIV/AIDS into the school curriculum

- Including HIV/AIDS in out-of-class activities (assemblies, home room time, anonymous school question boxes)

- Supporting co-curricular activities (school health clubs and information corners)

- Fostering peer support

- Involving the wider community.

Integrating and infusing teaching about HIV/AIDS into the school curriculum

The MoEST curriculum commits one period a week for teaching about HIV/AIDS. In addition, teachers work in groups to plan where, in their respective subjects, HIV/AIDS links can be found. Identification of links enables incorporation of MoEST's HIV/AIDS syllabus into classroom teaching throughout the curriculum, with teachers determining the methodology to be used to teach each topic identified.

Including HIV/AIDS in out-of-class activities

In many schools more than half of HIV/AIDS messages are conveyed during home-room time. Anonymous question boxes have also been found to be effective. Each week trained teachers respond to the questions submitted, clarifying conflicting messages and addressing cultural issues that may lead to the spread of HIV. Use of the boxes has been shown to break the silence surrounding not only HIV but also sexuality issues.

Young peoples' voices about the Question Box

Young people in classes 7 and 8 usually hold meetings once in a while. We talk about the problems we have encountered. We receive the answers to the questions written by students and put in the question box. Quite often the questions are so sensitive that students do not feel free to go directly to the teacher to ask the question. For instance, one girl writes that she is worried because she has never menstruated. She wonders whether she is abnormal. Some questions have been written by girls who are too scared or shy to tell their mothers that their stepfathers want to sleep with them. They fear becoming pregnant and being infected with STDs and HIV.

Female student, 15 years old

Supporting co-curricular activities

Channeling messages through various aspects of extracurricular activities, such as drama, debating clubs, song, and dance, helps ensure that the program follows a whole-school approach. School health clubs are also important in transmitting health messages.

Fostering peer support

Peer supporters trained by the program speak directly to students about personal concerns related to family, relationships, sex, and condoms. They help young people deal with pressures to be sexually active. In addition to functioning within and around the school environment, peer supporters play important roles in extracurricular activities.

Involving the wider community

The program aims to enable the wider community to recognize its role in partnership with schools in preventing the spread of HIV. It seeks to enable adults to deliver accurate and effective information about the transmission, prevention, and management of HIV. It encourages adults to lead and support young people in behavior change, get more involved in young people's activities, become stronger role models, protect the rights of children, and speak out against abuse.

The program provides a starting point and encourages a combined response from the community. It is not, however, able to provide resources to encourage community responses on any scale.

Implementation

A key feature of PSABH has been its ability rapidly to expand to a large number of schools without loss of quality in delivery of its interventions. This achievement is the product of a number of factors.

Partnerships

Strong coordination at the national, regional, district, and local levels has enabled PSABH partners to bring their respective strengths to HIV prevention in schools. MoEST coordinates the development of relevant policies, creating the necessary space for inclusion of HIV/AIDS education, prevention, and mitigation in the regular curriculum. It also conducts PSABH training sessions and facilitates the monitoring and evaluation of the program. CfBT is responsible for the daily management of the program. KIE's teaching-learning materials are used in the program. The Ministry of Health supports training, with ministry trainers facilitating PSABH training sessions as well as providing additional support to the teaching-learning taking place in schools.

Management Structure

Maintenance of a high-quality, full-scale intervention has demanded a strong and effective management structure. The Ministry of Education provides coordination officers in each region. These staff are involved in working groups and sensitization programs.

Sensitization meetings are held with key stakeholders, including education personnel at the provincial, district, zonal, and school levels; tribal chiefs; mayors; District Health Officers; and representatives of the district commissioners and other agencies working in HIV prevention. During meetings the program is introduced, coverage discussed, and selection criteria of schools and people to be involved determined. Logistics and responsibilities are agreed on, and trainers' selection criteria are endorsed.

Training

Training is an ongoing process for the program. Continual training is essential to maintain program coverage, quality, and succession. It is a time-consuming but critical activity.

PSABH has adopted a model of training that it refers to as a "strengthened cascade" (figure 6.2). This model has worked well in scaling the program up.[3] Members of the "lead" PSABH team (including program staff,

Figure 6.2: Coordinated Training Model of the Primary School Action for Better Health Program

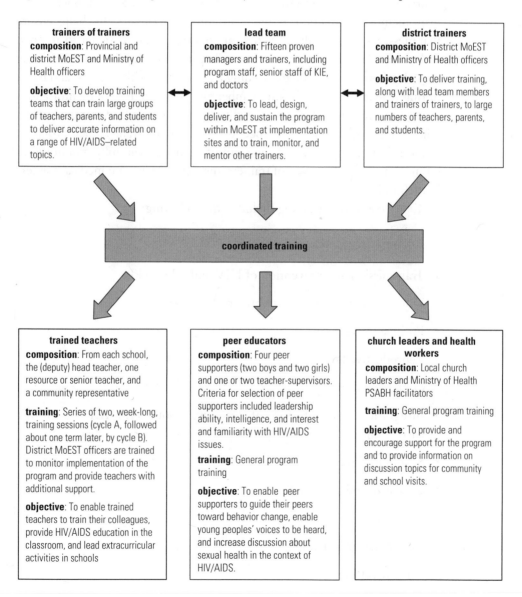

trainers of trainers
composition: Provincial and district MoEST and Ministry of Health officers

objective: To develop training teams that can train large groups of teachers, parents, and students to deliver accurate information on a range of HIV/AIDS–related topics.

lead team
composition: Fifteen proven managers and trainers, including program staff, senior staff of KIE, and doctors

objective: To lead, design, deliver, and sustain the program within MoEST at implementation sites and to train, monitor, and mentor other trainers.

district trainers
composition: District MoEST and Ministry of Health officers

objective: To deliver training, along with lead team members and trainers of trainers, to large numbers of teachers, parents, and students.

coordinated training

trained teachers
composition: From each school, the (deputy) head teacher, one resource or senior teacher, and a community representative

training: Series of two, week-long, training sessions (cycle A, followed about one term later, by cycle B). District MoEST officers are trained to monitor implementation of the program and provide teachers with additional support.

objective: To enable trained teachers to train their colleagues, provide HIV/AIDS education in the classroom, and lead extracurricular activities in schools

peer educators
composition: Four peer supporters (two boys and two girls) and one or two teacher-supervisors. Criteria for selection of peer supporters included leadership ability, intelligence, and interest and familiarity with HIV/AIDS issues.

training: General program training

objective: To enable peer supporters to guide their peers toward behavior change, enable young peoples' voices to be heard, and increase discussion about sexual health in the context of HIV/AIDS.

church leaders and health workers
composition: Local church leaders and Ministry of Health PSABH facilitators

training: General program training

objective: To provide and encourage support for the program and to provide information on discussion topics for community and school visits.

senior staff of KIE, and a team of doctors) train "trainers of trainers" drawn from district and provincial offices of MoEST and the Ministry of Health. Trainers of trainers are responsible in provinces for the formation of teams capable of training large groups of teachers, peer educators, church leaders, and health workers to deliver accurate information on a range of HIV-related topics. The lead team also trains district trainers, drawn from MoEST and Ministry of Health district offices, who support the work of the "trainers of trainers" at the district level. Training of trainers and training of district trainers usually takes about two weeks. Training of teachers, peer educators, church leaders, and health workers is always attended by a set number of lead team members, trainers of trainers, and district trainers. This helps ensure that messages are not diluted as they are passed from one trainer to another. At least one lead team member must take part in all training events, playing the role of overall coordinator, leading daily reviews with trainers, and monitoring delivery. The lead team member also plays the role of mentor and is expected to coach trainers of trainers to become future lead team members. The training guidelines also specify the ratios of trainers per group of trainees. The composition of the team of trainers is carefully monitored to ensure a mixture of trainers of trainers, district trainers, and medical trainers in each training team.

Topics covered in training included the following:

- School planning for health

- Transmission and prevention of HIV and other STIs

- Voluntary counseling and treatment

- Positive living

- Reproductive health

- Home-based care

- Integration and infusion of teaching about HIV/AIDS into the curriculum

- School health clubs

- Guidance and counseling

- Sexuality

- Co-curricular activities

- Climate setting

- Child rights

- Curriculum overview

- Question boxes

- Adolescent health

- Life skills

- Sexuality

- Emerging issues

Team members also receive training on:

- training techniques

- financial management, record keeping, and reporting

- team work

- management of materials

- micro-teaching

- development of Knowledge, Attitude, and Practice (KAP).

During teacher training, trainers use the same kinds of teaching-learning methods and activities that teachers will be expected to apply during their lessons. Like classroom activities, training is participatory, allowing teachers to see how the activities are done and experience different active learning methods and activities themselves.

In addition to training team members, the program trains selected district education officers, who are expected to monitor program implementation and provide support to teachers. Deans of Kenya's 28 primary teacher training colleges also receive training, in the form of a two-week program that focuses on incorporating HIV/AIDS education into the teacher training program.

Community members attend most of the same sessions as teachers. When teachers work on lesson planning, community members attend other sessions (dealing with community mobilization, for example).

Curricular Approach and Time Allocation

The program uses a combination of curricular approaches:

- HIV/AIDS is taught in a main carrier subject (in place of one weekly physical education lesson).

- HIV/AIDS is integrated into courses on health science, religious education, and social studies.

- HIV/AIDS is infused into the remainder of the curriculum.

- HIV/AIDS is taught through co-curricular and extracurricular activities.

Except for the one hour a week spent during physical education class, the amount of time devoted to HIV during the weekly timetable is not specified. Time allocation differs from school to school.

Materials

Development of program materials has been an ongoing activity, with the results of research and the insights and understanding of program managers and implementers incorporated into materials over time. Qualitative and quantitative research carried out at the start of the program provided critical information on students' sociocultural environment and the pressures and difficulties they face. This information fed into the development of both program and training materials.

Teacher materials

Members of the PSABH management team and program implementers, including MoEST, the Ministry of Health, and KIE, developed project-specific manuals and handbooks for the program. The materials take students through behavior change–related sessions. The first materials produced (PSABH Module A) cover the following topics:

- Kenya's goals for education

- HIV/AIDS syllabus and recommended approaches, methodologies, and materials

- Information about HIV/AIDS

- Life-skills and living-values education and approaches

- Roles of guidance and counseling

- Integration and infusion of teaching about HIV/AIDS into the curriculum

- Use of in-class and out-of-class time and methodologies

- Emerging issues

- School and community response.

In the initial design of the program, participants returned for a second week of training after one semester back at school. Module B materials were developed to revisit the initial training material, with tighter focus on the needs of young people and the need for interactive teaching methods. Over time the two modules were merged into a single training publication.

Project materials are supplemented by publications such as *The AIDS Handbook* and *Choices: A Guide for Young People*.

Young people and conflicting HIV messages

Parents should be actively involved. They should not be shy but should be actively involved in educating their children about HIV/AIDS. The government and particularly the Minister for Health should openly talk about HIV/AIDS to children and adults. Pastors too should teach about the subject.

Female peer supporter, 13 years old

The condom message for instance is confusing. The government recommends that people use the condom. Often teachers and Churches say the opposite, that we should not use condoms.

Female peer supporter, 13 years old

Classroom materials

The program used a range of classroom materials for different ages and activities:

- *Let's Talk about AIDS* books, developed by KIE, available as class sets in schools for use at the teachers' discretion

- HIV/AIDS readers (short-story books depicting how HIV/AIDS affects people's lives and how the people in the stories respond)

- Videos, such as "Silent Epidemic" and "Everyone's Child"; materials from The AIDS Support Organization (TASO) on HIV/AIDS counseling; and the "Bush Fire" and "Sara" materials

- *Stay Alive* materials (an eight-week course for children in classes 4 and 5, including discussion of topics with parents

- "Family impact" lesson plans and teaching resources, for classes 7 and 8, including a component that engages parents

- Additional resources provided by a range of stakeholders, including the Red Cross, the Child Welfare Society of Kenya, and the Ministry of Health AIDS Control Unit.

Peer-supporter materials

Peer-supporter materials prepared by PSABH working groups are used during training and in schools as reference materials. The materials seek to help peer supporters help young people make informed choices about relationships and sexual behavior through skills and values development.

School health club kit

Every participating school receives a school health club kit that covers:

- life skills, living values, and related activities
- goal setting
- school health activities
- HIV/AIDS management
- dealing with external conflicting messages through song and dance
- love and sex
- setting one's own agenda.

They also receive a question box that enables students anonymously to post questions to be answered by teachers during class discussions.

Evaluation

Evaluation and research are essential parts of PSABH. They have enabled continuous review of program activities and objectives to ensure that measurable impact is being made. According to program manager Mary Gichuru, "Many programs deliver a 'package' that has been designed at the beginning and is the same at the end. Staff are not always encouraged or supported to adapt material in the light of changing circumstances and information. Programs can develop only if they have mechanisms to respond and adapt."

An important part of the rationale underlying the program has been the belief that activities must start with detailed knowledge of the risks of HIV infection from the perspective of the young person, including information about how risks start, develop, proceed, and can be avoided. Information is also needed about the problems and challenges that those charged with delivering prevention materials may face.

For HIV education to be effective, full knowledge of the culturally specific factors affecting both transmission and the delivery of health messages is vital. Well-researched, up-to-date knowledge is particularly important in a time of rapid cultural change.

PSABH was based on an understanding of the culture in which Kenyan children and teachers live. It also reflects understanding of how education

---

HIV education in a changing cultural context

Traditionally, discussing sex openly was taboo. Grandparents, however, advised the youth about cultural norms and taught them that sex was 'sacred.' The interaction between communities and the outside culture has since changed this culture. The media also played a great part in change.

PSABH lead trainer

Messages delivered need to be clear, honest and consistent. Young people are particularly attuned to picking up a range of views as they try to develop their own characters and ways in society. Unless messages are consistent with those of other key players such as politicians, religious leaders and media personalities, it is more difficult to achieve a sustained impact.

PSABH manager

---

works in Kenya, how schools work, how the education system functions, and how schooling forms and modifies behavior.

Research conducted at all stages of the program has enabled constant attention to be paid to the knowledge, attitudes, and behavior of school-age children in Kenya; the course of the HIV epidemic; and the impact of the program. Such attention has led to continuing evolution of the aims, nature, and delivery of activities to ensure their maximum impact in preventing HIV infection. Research has also been important in helping advocates push for continuance and expansion of the program. It has shown skeptics that their fears of the program were unwarranted.

Methodology

Methods used for data collection included self-completed questionnaires (completed by head teachers and students); in-depth interviews (of teachers and community members); focus group discussions (of students); and surveys of school and community responsiveness (based on zonal inspectors' visits). Data were collected before the program was introduced, 14–18 months after teachers were trained, and 26–30 months after training.[4] The evaluation surveyed 10,000 students, 700 head teachers and teachers, and 68 local leaders and community representatives. It included 116 schools in which PSABH was in place and 62 control schools.

The survey and interviews focused on the following issues:

- Knowledge about transmission and prevention of HIV

- Attitudes toward risk and prevention

- Teaching and activities in school

- Sexual behavior (students only)

- Attitudes toward sexual, gender, and cultural issues
- Community behavior and activities.

Results

At 18 months the program showed the following impressive results in target schools (table 6.1):

- Sexual initiation among both boys and girls was delayed.
- Fewer boys and girls reported they had ever had sex.
- More girls reported having been forced to have sex.
- More boys reported avoiding places in order not to have sex.
- More girls reported condom use during last sexual encounter.
- More girls felt they could say no to sex.
- More girls believed that "no" means "no."
- More girls and boys felt they could have a boyfriend and girlfriend and not have sex.
- More boys and girls felt they could tell their boyfriend or girlfriend that the preferred to wait until marriage before having sex.

Table 6.1: Odds Ratios for Impact of Interventions on Student Behavior and Attitudes

ITEM	BOYS	GIRLS
Ever had sex	0.80**	0.86**
Had first sexual experience in past year	0.62***	0.60***
Ever forced to have sex	0.90	1.15*
Ever avoided a place to avoid sex	1.35**	1.07
Used condom during last sexual encounter	1.07	1.53**
Can definitely say no to sex	1.07	1.30**
Can definitely have a boyfriend or girlfriend and not have sex	1.20*	1.30**
Can definitely tell boyfriend or girlfriend that I prefer to wait until I am married to have sex	1.15*	1.25**
Definitely believe "no" means "no"	0.90	1.20**

Source: CfBT.

* Significant at the 5 percent level. ** Significant at the 1 percent level. *** Significant at the 0.1 percent level.

Note: Odds ratios compare the size of the changes among the student population in the target schools and those in control schools, taking account of the baseline difference between the target and control groups. An odds ratio of 1 represents no difference between target and control schools, a ratio greater than 1 represents an increase in target schools, and a ratio less than 1 represents a decrease in target schools. The farther the ratio is from 1, the larger the change. An odds ratio of 0.60 for girls' sexual initiation indicates that the net gain in delaying first sexual encounter in the year before data collection for girls in target schools compared with control schools is 37.5 percent.

Eighteen months after the introduction of the program, there was no significant increase in the likelihood of students receiving a passing grade on the PSABH knowledge test, and there were no significant differences over time between target and control schools on either teacher or student knowledge (the odds ratios were 1.04 for students and 1.10 for teachers). In a subsequent evaluation, conducted 30 months postprogram, the difference was highly significant. Program implementation was also higher but student participation was slightly lower. The decline in student participation resulted from reduced use of question boxes and school health clubs. This change occurred as a result of the loss of trained teachers and peer supporters and the inclusion of HIV/AIDS activities in the programs of other school clubs.

Qualitative findings back up the results of quantitative research. Focus group discussions indicated dramatic shifts in students' abilities to describe concrete methods they used to avoid or refuse sex. They also revealed an increase in the accuracy and breadth of knowledge about HIV/AIDS.

At all waves of data collection, teachers and community leaders presented abstinence as the only truly effective method of preventing HIV infection. Over time teachers gradually incorporated specific teaching strategies to help students abstain from sex and increase their sense of personal control and efficacy in sexual decision making. Schools also invited outsiders, such as health workers and staff of local NGOs, to discuss how condoms help prevent HIV transmission.

Thirty months after training, students and teachers listed more reasons for abstaining from sex in order to avoid HIV infection and death than they

---

Changes in teaching

Initially teachers taught:

- *'HIV/AIDS kills'*
- *'It has no cure'*
- *'You must abstain'*

With training they now teach:

- *'This is how you can abstain from early sex'*
- *'There are many reasons why you should abstain'*
- *'If you really can't abstain, you should use a condom'* (for those whom the teacher thinks are sexually active)

The messages teachers now give the children include:

- *'Sex is for married people'*
- *'Sex is sacred'*
- *'Early sex is harmful to your health'*

did before the program or 18 months after training. In addition, although teachers focus on persuading students to abstain from sex rather than use condoms, there appeared to be an increase in the discussion of condom use to prevent HIV.

The effectiveness of six models was tested:

- *Basic model.* The head teacher, one teacher, and one community representative from each school received five days of training (six nights of accommodation) in cycle A and four days (five nights of accommodation) in cycle B (provided about one term after cycle A).

- *Church leader model.* In addition to the basic model, each school was invited to send a local church leader to the same training. All four school representatives trained together.

- *Health worker model.* Trainers from the Ministry of Health who had been trained as PSABH facilitators received extra briefings on visiting schools and were given a list of topics to cover. Modest funds were provided for each facilitator to make three visits to a school to talk to students on the agreed-upon topics.

- *Additional teachers model.* In addition to the basic model, each school was invited to send two other teachers for training. These teachers were trained after the core team was trained.

- *Peer supporter model.* In addition to the basic model, schools were invited to send four Standard 6 or 7 students, along with one teacher, to attend three days of training (four nights of accommodation).

- *Cost-share model.* Participating schools bore the cost of travel, accommodations, and board of their three participants.

The evaluation yielded several interesting findings:

- The different models produced few significant differences in outcomes. The differences that did exist suggested that training additional teachers was the most effective variant.

- Health workers and church leaders visited schools under all variations. However, they visited significantly more schools when they were specifically directed to. Health workers visited more than 90 percent of schools in the health worker variation; church leaders visited 71 percent in their variation. The topics discussed and the messages brought by health workers and church leaders were not influenced by PSABH training: both made abstinence the dominant prevention message. In the minority of cases where health workers spoke about condoms, they provided information and addressed individual questions. Church leaders placed abstinence within a religious and cultural context, providing biblical and faith-based reasons for abstaining rather than focusing on fear of HIV.

- Peer supporters were well received by students and teachers alike and had a positive impact on both the level of school programming and student knowledge, attitudes, and beliefs. Students rated peer supporters highly on all characteristics and tasks. Peer supporters were better able than teachers to speak directly to students about their concerns related to family, sex, boyfriends/girlfriends, condoms, and pressures to be sexually active. Selection of peer supporters who can provide the best role models with respect to sexual activity is important. Students question when peer supporters say one thing and do another.

Cost-Effectiveness

An important feature of the project design was the ability to follow the cost and effectiveness of activities, in particular to track the cost and impact of different variations in training used (table 6.2).

For all models except the cost-share model, costs included the following components (table 6.3):

- Round-trip transportation to workshops for each participant

- Full-board accommodation for participants in dormitories at teacher training colleges or similar venues

Table 6.2: Distribution of Project Costs in Nyanza Region

ITEM	PERCENTAGE OF TOTAL SPENDING
Project component	
Design, printing, and distributing school teaching-learning materials	22
School and community training	15
Personnel	15
Capacity building of trainers	10
Research	10
Training of peer supporters	8
Offices	7
Equipment	4
Sensitization of schools not included in program activities	3
Mobilization/field planning	2
Training at teacher training colleges	1
Development of training materials	1
MoEST liaison	1
Kenyan technical advisers	1

Source: CfBT.

Table 6.3: Program Costs, by Training Model
(U.S. dollars)

MODEL	PER SCHOOL	PER ADULT	PER STUDENT
Basic PSABH	360	120	3.00
Church leader	479	120	3.99
Health worker visits	488	n.a.	4.06
Additional teachers	603	120	5.03
Peer supporter	758	n.a.	6.30
Cost-share	90	30	0.76

Source: CfBT.
n.a. Not applicable.
Note: Costs show the marginal cost of the program. They do not include the cost of the set of KIE texts provided to each school (about $192 per box).

- Stationery and handouts for each workshop

- One set of KIE texts per participant (HIV/AIDS syllabus, book III of *Let's Talk about AIDS*, and *Facilitator's Handbook*)

- Round-trip transportation to workshops for facilitators

- Full-board accommodation for facilitators

- Per diem allowances for facilitators.

Modifying the Program in Response to Research

The use of research enabled the messages, methods, and training employed by the program to be amended and optimized over time. Issues to which research drew attention included gender, sexual activity, teachers' ability to deliver education, Kenya's changing culture, and cost-effectiveness.

Gender issues

Research on the sexual experience of young people in Kenya facilitated development of an understanding of the fact that sexual encounters are typically the end result of a sequence of events that begins with expression of interest (typically by a boy). Research highlighted the importance of providing gender-specific education about sexuality and HIV/AIDS. In response the program began to deliver education to girls- and boys-only groups.

Sexual activity

As the program was implemented, it became apparent that a large percentage of upper-primary school students were already sexually active. In response to this realization, the program introduced a broader range of prevention messages and strategies, not only targeting the needs of students yet to become sexual active but also trying to change the behaviors of those already having sex. Program materials were modified to provide more objective information about prevention and concrete strategies for abstinence.

Teachers' ability to deliver education

Operational research conducted for the program revealed differences in the way that trained personnel were interpreting and delivering the program materials. It became apparent that adults' belief systems made them uncomfortable in delivering some areas of knowledge and skills to younger children. Training was modified to enable teachers to overcome their discomfort.

Kenya's changing culture

Research demonstrated the ways in which poverty drives some young people in Kenya to engage in prostitution or to exchange sex for goods provided by "sugar daddies." Cultural factors such as wife inheritance and early marriage can also act to increase the risks of transmission. Gender expectations can lead many young people, especially girls, to feel that they are forced into sex. In response to these findings, the program was modified to strengthen its ability to enable students to make healthy choices in the difficult environments in which many live. Changes included enabling guidance and counseling teachers to assist with peer support training, encouraging the participation of church leaders in training, and helping college lecturers to disseminate AIDS information to college students.

Cost-effectiveness

Several changes are recommended based on the cost-effectiveness assessment of the program:

- The number of teachers trained per school should be increased by two, so that each school trains one head teacher, three teachers, and one community representative for five days (six nights' accommodation).

- A team of three (one head teacher, one teacher, and one community representative) should be trained first, with additional teachers trained one semester later in workshops created entirely for teachers.

- Five church leaders from the three dominant churches plus two local churches should be invited to each workshop.

Table 6.4: Estimated Costs of Revised PSABH Training Package
(U.S. dollars)

COMPONENT	PER SCHOOL	PER ADULT	PER STUDENT
Revised PSABH model	381	76	3.18
Revised peer support	696	n.a.	5.79

Source: CfBT.
n.a. Not applicable.

- Some schools should be invited to send four Standard 6 or 7 students, along with one teacher, to attend four days' (accommodation five nights) training. The number of schools sending peer supporters will depend on funding and timing as adults need to be trained first to create a suitable and supportive environment for student peer supporters.

Making these changes is projected to raise the cost of the teaching program to $3.18 per student and reduce the cost of peer support to $5.79 per student (table 6.4).

Lessons Learned

The PSABH program encountered a wide range of challenges and has learned many lessons. The lessons described here are based on interviews with program managers and implementers.

Dealing with Turnover

Turnover among teachers and peer educators was high: 22 percent of schools lost trained teachers to transfer or death during an 18-month period. Replacing graduating peer supporters presented enormous difficulties. As a result, the program decided not to continue primary-level peer support in order to maximize sustainability.

Conveying Consistent Messages

Research highlighted young people's sensitivity to the range of messages they hear about HIV/AIDS from parents, teachers, religious leaders, the media, and other sources. Experience gained in the program showed that prevention is most effective when messages delivered are conveyed consistently by a wide range of sources.

School visits by trained health workers were found to be helpful in discussing sensitive topics, such as prevention of infection. The use of peer educators improved the nature and level of communication on HIV risk. Participation of religious leaders increased awareness of the need for consistent messages.

The program stresses the benefits of separating objective information from moral education on sexual issues, emphasizing that accurate information alone does not promote earlier or more frequent sexual activity. Lack of ability to provide clear messages about condoms presents a clear challenge for the program. The MoEST curriculum is silent about condoms and their use; the policy about condoms in school is "no promotion, distribution or demonstration." Lessons on condom use are not part of the program, although training covers condom use. Teachers are, however, allowed to answer questions students raise about condoms, and they may respond to questions posed at school health clubs or through question boxes. Research shows that young people appreciate receiving accurate information as they struggle to create a complete understanding of HIV risk and prevention.

Ensuring Sustainability

The program aims to develop sustainable systems that will continue even when no external body manages the program. To keep costs low, it does not pay per diem allowances for training; attendees receive full-board accommodations and reimbursement for travel expenses. The high quality of training usually means that those attending accept these conditions. Trainers receive some small allowances for delivering training. Reducing reliance on per diem allowances ensures that those who work for the program do so out of their own sense of social, professional, and personal commitment rather than desire for financial return.

The wisdom of a program manager

- Listen to the needs of young people
- Respect the difficulties adults have
- Work to meet both of the above
- Remain flexible enough to allow communities to prioritize their needs and develop their own solutions
- Build research as an integral part of the program
- Manage the training team with expertise – keep the content tight and consistent
- Give clear, complete, manageable prevention messages
- Check what messages are being received as well as delivered
- Involve the appropriate levels of the ministry at the beginning and continue a dialogue giving feedback of research findings
- Don't provide pre-packaged manuals early on – they stop people from thinking for themselves

Avoiding Message Diffusion

Some implementers believe that teachers have too little time to address HIV/AIDS–related issues in depth. Some teachers were reluctant to teach about HIV/AIDS because it felt like a burden. In some cases the high pupil-teacher ratio limited interactions between teacher and students.

The broad integration and use of different curricular approaches is a strength of the approach in Kenya, in that it allows for many entry points for teaching and learning about HIV/AIDS. It may also lead to diffusion, however.

If schools or districts have some flexibility in curriculum delivery, it could be worthwhile assessing how much additional time is required to teach about HIV/AIDS–related issues and to provide schools with support in revising parts of the curriculum to create time and space for teaching-learning about HIV/AIDS. Program implementers suggest that making the subject examinable would encourage teachers to teach it and students to take it more seriously.

Conclusions

The PSABH program provides high-quality education on HIV prevention to thousands of children across Kenya. Its success can be related to a number of factors:

- The use of upper-primary schools as the locus for activities, enabling the majority of children in a community to be reached

- Inclusion of a range of key stakeholders providing political will, curriculum expertise, and management efficiency

- Employment of a management and training structure that allows quality to be maintained in the face of rapid expansion

- The use of well-designed research to hone program approaches and document the program's impact

- The use of well-researched training materials and continuing attention to high-quality training

- Attention to sustainability, by ensuring that motivation for participation comes from social and personal commitment rather than reliance on financial reward.

Annex 6.1

PSABH Attainment of Impact Benchmarks

BENCHMARK	ATTAINMENT/COMMENTS
1. Identifies and focuses on specific sexual health goals	✓ The program is highly focused on the transmission and prevention of HIV and on enabling students to take control of their own sexual lives and avoid infection.
2. Focuses narrowly on specific behaviors that lead to sexual health goals	Partial. The program focused on promotion of abstinence and the creation of strong and effective and faithful relationships. Teaching on use of condoms was not clear due to the personal and professional challenges faced by teachers.
3. Identifies and focuses on sexual psychosocial risk and protective factors that are highly related to each of these behaviors	✓ The program focused on enabling students to take control of their own sexual lives teaching strategies such as avoiding risky places and behaviors, how to say no, and so forth.
4. Implements multiple activities to change each of the selected risk and protective factors	✓ The program used a wide range of strategies, including teaching in different areas, school health clubs, peer educators, outreach to the community, and so forth.
5. Actively involves youth by creating a safe social environment	✓ Gender- and age-sensitive teaching, the use of anonymous question boxes, use of peer educators, etc. all led to creation of a safe social environment for participation.
6. Employs a variety of teaching methods designed to involve participants and have them personalize the information	✓ A wide variety of participatory teaching methodologies was used to teach the program curriculum.
7. Conveys clear message about sexual activity and condom or contraceptive use and continually reinforces that message	Partial. See benchmark 2.
8. Includes effective curricula and activities appropriate to the age, sexual experience, and culture of participating students	✓ Highly effective research ensured that curricula and messages were tailored to the circumstances and lived reality of students.
9. Increases knowledge by providing basic, accurate information about the risks of teen sexual activity and methods of avoiding intercourse or using protection against pregnancy and STIs	✓ Course content concerning knowledge about HIV was strong and clear.
10. Uses some of the same strategies to change perceptions of peer values, to recognize peer pressure to have sex, and to address that pressure	✓ Impact assessments showed that use of peer educators was particularly effective in helping peer issues to be addressed.
11. Identifies specific situations that might lead to sex, unwanted sex, or unprotected sex and identifies methods of avoiding those situations or getting out of them	✓ Role-plays, dramas, and anonymous question boxes enabled students to identify situations that might lead to sex and their avoidance.
12. Provides modeling of and practice with communication, negotiation, and refusal skills to improve both skills and self-efficacy in using those skills.	✓ The life-skills content of curriculum encouraged students to learn and use communication, negotiation, and refusal skills.

Source: Authors.

Annex 6.2

Contact Information

Centre for British Teachers
12th Floor
IPS Building
Kimathi St.
Nairobi, Kenya
Mailing address: P.O. BOX 45774, 01001 Nairobi
Tel: +254 20 252121/226917
Fax: +254 20 305411
E-mail: jwildish@cfbtken.co.ke
Web site: www.psabh.info

Notes

1. Children in Kenya spend seven years of primary schooling, usually beginning at age 7. Secondary schooling usually begins at age 14 and lasts five years. Some older children (over 14 years) may be in primary education owing to having started school later than at 7 years.

2. CfBT is a not-for-profit organization funded by the Department for International Development. It manages education sector projects all over the world. Its Nairobi office has provided management assistance to several national education sector interventions since its opening in 1992.

3. There is continual turnover, especially in the groups of trainers of trainers and district trainers. This turnover is one of the reasons why the program needs to ensure that training is ongoing.

4. It was not possible to use the same control sites in the second phase of the evaluation, because the schools were promised training following completion of the 18-month evaluation.

Primary School AIDS Prevention at a Glance

Description: The Ministry of Education, Science, and Technology (MoEST) and an NGO, the International Child Support (ICS), collaborated on the implementation of four approaches aimed at reducing risky behavior among adolescents in the Western Province of Kenya. The different approaches were offered in groups to randomly selected schools, creating a unique opportunity rigorously to evaluate the impact of each.

Number of schools participating: 328

Coverage: Bungoma and Butere-Mumias District, Western Province, Kenya

Target group: Upper-primary students in public schools (ages 12–16)

Components: The program consisted of four interventions: teacher training, debates and essay-writing contests, a lecture on the dangers of cross-generational sex, and provision of free school uniforms

Establishment and duration: 2003–05

Management: ICS

Role of MoEST: Teacher training and implementation of programs in schools

Role of partners: The Abdul Latif Jameel Poverty Action Lab at the Massachusetts Institute of Technology assisted with program design and conducted monitoring and evaluation. The Partnership for Child Development and the World Bank provided funding.

Costs: Teacher training to improve delivery of HIV/AIDS curriculum cost $408 per school, $146 per teacher, and $2 per student. Promotion of active learning through debates and essay writing cost $109 per school and $1.10 per student. Warning adolescents about the dangers of cross-generational sex cost $28 per school and $0.80 per student. Providing free school uniforms cost $12 per student.

Key evaluation results: Teacher training increased the amount of time devoted to the HIV/AIDS curriculum, had no impact on teenage childbearing rates, increased the likelihood that girls who had started childbearing were married to the fathers of their children, promoted active learning through debates and essay writing, increased students' knowledge, and increased the likelihood of boys reporting having used condoms. Warning adolescents about the dangers of cross-generational sex reduced teenage childbearing. Providing free school uniforms increased school retention rates and reduced teenage childbearing and marriage rates.

The Primary School AIDS Prevention Program, Kenya

Although prevention of HIV is critical to control of the disease, little rigorous evidence from randomized studies about the relative effectiveness of different interventions has been produced. The effectiveness of scalable school-based HIV/AIDS education programs is also a subject of debate, with skeptics doubting both whether teachers can be effective and whether school-based prevention programs represent the best use of scarce prevention funds. There is also intense debate over the content of prevention programs, particularly whether condom use should be discussed.

In a review of 11 school-based HIV/AIDS education programs in Africa, Gallant and Maticka-Tyndale (2004) found that while most programs succeeded in improving knowledge and attitudes, the majority of programs failed to change behavior. Evaluations that claim a change in behavior often rely on self-reported data to assess their impact. But self-reported data may suffer from social desirability biases, in which students report the behavior they think is "right" rather than their actual conduct.

Description

The Primary School AIDS Prevention Program used a randomized study designed to evaluate the impact of four approaches for reducing risky behavior among adolescents in Kenya's Western Province. Researchers measured the effects of the interventions on young people's knowledge about, attitudes toward, and reported practice of sex; rates of teen pregnancy and early marriage; and retention in school. They also estimated the costs of the four

Pascaline Dupas, assistant professor of economics at Dartmouth College and member of the Abdul Latif Jameel Poverty Action Lab at the Massachusetts Institute of Technology (MIT), and Willa Friedman, evaluation consultant at the Abdul Latif Jameel Poverty Action Lab at MIT, prepared this chapter. Michael Kremer provided support, encouragement, and assistance.

interventions. The results will enable policy makers and program managers to make informed decisions.

Rationale and History

A survey conducted in Western Kenya in 2002 suggested that the extent to which the country's HIV/AIDS curriculum was being taught was worrisomely low. In response, the National AIDS Control Council (NACC) and Ministry of Education, Science, and Technology (MoEST) hosted a consultation with officials from MoEST, NACC, the Kenya Institute of Education (KIE), the Center for British Teachers (CfBT), the World Bank, International Child Support (ICS), and academics. Four key concerns were identified.

Poor implementation of the HIV/AIDS curriculum

Kenya's primary-school national AIDS curriculum and textbooks were developed in 1999 by KIE, an arm of MoEST, with assistance from UNICEF and extensive input from civic and religious groups in Kenya. The 2002 survey of Western Kenya revealed that despite the introduction of the facilitator's handbook to all primary schools, effective teaching of HIV/AIDS in schools was sporadic. Other than receiving the handbook, the vast majority of teachers had not received guidance or training on how to impart HIV/AIDS education to their students. Visits to schools and classroom observations suggested that many schools were not providing HIV/AIDS education, often because teachers did not feel comfortable or competent to teach the subject. In schools that did provide lessons on HIV/AIDS, not all teachers conveyed accurate information.

In an effort to address these shortcomings, MoEST hired trainers to provide in-service courses for teachers on HIV/AIDS education based on the techniques in the facilitator's handbook. Because of budget constraints, only a few teachers were offered this training.

Lack of engagement with HIV/AIDS issues

Rather than encourage students to engage with the material and the issues raised, HIV/AIDS education often merely provides information. Participants at the meeting expressed the need to encourage students to remember more about what is discussed in class and to think critically about what they hear, in order to be able to put what they know into practice.

The dangers of cross-generational sex

Cross-generational sex is associated with an increased risk of HIV infection for adolescent girls, because HIV prevalence among men increases with age. "Sugar daddies"—older men who provide adolescent girls with gifts in return for sex—represent a significant risk. Because such relationships are common, women 15–19 are significantly more likely than men their age to be infected with HIV.

Financial barriers to girls' education

Although school fees were abolished in Kenya in 2003, financial barriers to education at the primary level remain. One of the most important is the cost of school uniforms, which, at a cost of about $6, represent a substantial expense for parents in a country where in 2004, average per capita GNI was $460 (UNICEF 2006). Schools are supposed to admit students whether or not they wear a uniform, but this rule is not always followed. Moreover, even when students without uniforms are admitted to school, they are likely to feel embarrassed that their peers know that their families are poor.

The impact of financial barriers on girls' participation in education is of particular concern, because retention of girls in schools is considered vital to HIV prevention. Staying in school may induce girls to delay sexual activity or to use contraception, for a variety of reasons. First, the value of abstinence and delayed childbearing is taught in schools. Second, because girls who become pregnant typically face strong social pressure to leave school (although they are entitled legally to attend), reducing the cost of education raises the opportunity cost of pregnancy and thus of unprotected sex. More generally, by increasing a woman's human capital and earning power, education increases the opportunity cost of being pregnant.

The need to evaluate interventions

In response to these concerns, Kenya's MoEST decided that much more information was needed about different methods of HIV prevention if policy makers and program managers were to make informed decisions about activities. The ministry, along with a number of its partner agencies, worked with staff of the Abdul Latif Poverty Action Lab at the Massachusetts Institute of Technology (MIT) to design a robust study that would allow the impact of different interventions to be evaluated. Implementation was led by an NGO, International Child Support (ICS).

Aims and Objectives

The aim of the program was to reduce the spread of HIV among young people in Kenya and throughout Africa. The objectives of the program were twofold: to identify what works and what does not in reducing the transmission of HIV among young people and to encourage the widespread replication of successful strategies.

Target Group

All programs targeted upper-primary school students (12- to 16-year-old boys and girls enrolled in grades 5–8).

Implementation

Components

The program implemented and rigorously evaluated the effectiveness and cost-effectiveness of four interventions:

- Teacher training

- Debates and essay-writing contests

- A lecture on the dangers of cross-generational sex

- Provision of free school uniforms.

All of the interventions are inexpensive and replicable strategies for raising HIV awareness and encouraging safe sexual and reproductive behavior among young people living in resource-poor settings.

Teacher training

To enhance the delivery of the national HIV/AIDS education curriculum, in-service training was provided to 540 primary-school teachers from 175 schools in three districts of Western Province between September 2002 and June 2003. The training sessions were conducted jointly by the AIDS Control Unit of the Ministry of Education (ACU-MoEST), KIE, and ICS. They covered a wide range of topics, including basic facts on HIV/AIDS, a demonstration on condom use, information on voluntary counseling and testing, and a discussion of HIV/AIDS education methodology. The training was designed to equip teachers with tools that would help them integrate HIV/AIDS education into the subjects they taught, teach stand-alone lessons about HIV/AIDS, and help other teachers in their schools participate in HIV/AIDS education.

Each school was invited to send three teachers: the head teacher if possible and two other motivated teachers teaching upper-primary school, including at least one woman. Attendance at the training sessions was high, with 93 percent of those invited attending training.

The primary goal of the training was to provide teachers with the tools they needed to incorporate the government's HIV/AIDS education material into the primary-school curriculum. The training covered the same topics emphasized in the facilitator's handbook that had been distributed to all schools in Kenya, which covered

- facts about HIV/AIDS and other STIs,
- modes of HIV transmission,
- practices that promote the spread of HIV,
- prevention and control of HIV,
- support for people infected with and affected by HIV,
- social and economic consequences of HIV/AIDS,
- management of HIV/AIDS education activities in school,
- methods of teaching HIV/AIDS education,
- community involvement,
- infusion and integration of HIV/AIDS education into the curriculum,
- nutrition guidelines for people with HIV/AIDS, and
- gender issues, youth, and HIV/AIDS.

One of the training sessions was dedicated to the preparation of lesson plans for use in class. By the time teachers left, they had prepared at least 13 lessons, covering the following topics:

- What is HIV? What is AIDS?
- How does HIV spread?
- How does HIV not spread?
- How can boys be circumcised safely?
- Effects of AIDS on the body
- How to care for people living with AIDS
- How one can stay HIV free
- How to avoid sexually risky situations
- How to say no to sex
- Adolescence and sexuality
- Why students should delay sex
- What "safe sex" means
- How to advise friends and peers on sex issues and HIV prevention.

At the end of the training, teachers were asked to prepare an action plan for HIV/AIDS education in their school. Their plan included how they would reach out to other teachers and how they would integrate HIV/AIDS into the timetable.

ICS did not provide refresher courses. The nature of the relationship between ICS and the schools facilitated ongoing support for teachers, however. Each school was visited at least once per term to collect feedback.

In addition to delivering classroom-based activities, trained teachers were advised to set up health clubs to encourage HIV prevention through active learning activities, such as role-play. Health clubs were monitored through school visits. A year after the training, 86 percent of schools in which teachers had been trained had established health clubs. Trained teachers who had maintained active health clubs were given T-shirts with red ribbons and the message: "PAMOJA TUANGAMIZE UKIMWI" ("Together, let's crush AIDS"). Student members of the clubs received red ribbon pins to put on their school uniforms. Small grants of up to $50 were provided for health clubs that submitted proposals to organize HIV/AIDS awareness activities for youth in and out of school. In the first year, two-thirds of the schools submitted proposals that were approved.

Debating and essay writing

Debating is an established practice in Kenyan schools. In 2005, 82 schools were encouraged to organize debates among students in grades 7 and 8 on the motion "school children should be taught how to use condoms." This activity is recommended in the facilitator's handbook on HIV/AIDS education in primary schools, a manual prepared and distributed to all schools by KIE in collaboration with UNICEF. The debates were conducted in Swahili or English.

The same 82 schools were also invited to ask students in grades 7 and 8 to take part in an essay-writing competition on the topic "discuss ways in which you can protect yourself from HIV infection now and later in your life." Essays were written in English.

The purpose of the contest was to encourage students to think critically about the options available to them. All essays were collected by ICS. Teachers were asked not to read the essays before handing them over to ICS.

During the school break, ICS hired teachers from districts not included in the program, who graded the essays and selected the best essays written by a boy and a girl in each grade. The teachers were instructed to mark the essays based on their content and to reward the students with the most comprehensive plans for remaining HIV free. After the decisions were made, the four winners in each school were awarded school bags in a small ceremony at their schools, during which the best essay written in the district was read aloud. By publicly awarding two students per class, ICS identified knowledgeable students who could serve as resources to their classmates.

Some 9,500 students participated in the debating and essay-writing activities. Some excerpts from student essays are shown below.

> There are three ways; g protection. Absitenence Be faithful and use g condoms. If you don't follow these you will contract the virus and at long last you will die.

> That is why I made the following decisions to make sure that I remain permanently without AIDS.
> Firstly I will not have anything to do with boys before marriage.
> Secondly I shall make sure that I remain a virgin untill I get my future husband.
> Thirdly to make sure that the person I want to get married to, is without the disease, we shall first of all go to hospital for check-up.
> I shall be a faithful housewife to my husband and I shall encourage my husband also to be faithful.
> We shall be talking and I will tell my husband that if he cant manage to stay with me alone, he should be using condoms with other girls.

> You can be on your way home to school and then a rich man sees you and asks to give you a lift in his car. Oh! that man could be infected. So, I can protect myself from HIV/AIDS by avoid receiving gifts from people who are not my parents.

Sugar daddy talk

In 2004, 2,500 grade 8 students in 71 schools attended a 40-minute "sugar daddy talk," which informed them of the heightened risk of HIV infection associated with older men. The goal of the program was to help young people make more informed decisions by educating young women about the health risk associated with having sex with sugar daddies and educating young men about the health risk associated with having sex with classmates who are sexually involved with older men.

The lecture was conducted during the school day by a female field officer from ICS. To introduce the topic, the lecturer showed "Sara: The Trap," an educational video produced by UNICEF to warn young people about sugar daddies. (As most schools did not have electricity, ICS brought a small generator along with a TV and video cassette recorder to play the video.) After the presentation, the ICS facilitator conducted a brief discussion about the risk sugar daddies present to all students in the class. On the board she drew the following:

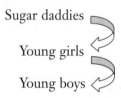

Sugar daddies

Young girls

Young boys

She then presented students with data on the age distribution of HIV in Kenya (table 7.1).

This information was followed by a second illustration of the risks:

HIV + sugar daddies

HIV + young girls

HIV + young boys

The field officer then conducted a brief question-and-answer session with students.

Free school uniforms

The program provided free school uniforms to 20,000 students. Students enrolled in grade 6 in 2003 were given one free uniform in the

Table 7.1: HIV Prevalence in Kisumu District, 1996

(percent)

ITEM	15–19	20–24	25–29	30–39
Men	4	13	29	24
Women	22	39	39	32

Source: Ministry of Health 2001.

spring of 2003 and a second 18 months later, provided they remained enrolled in the same school. ICS recruited local tailors, who visited the schools to take the measurements of all students eligible for free uniforms. They typically needed about a month to complete the uniforms for a given school.

Curricular Approach and Time Allocation

The program used a mix of interventions, two of which involved education of learners on HIV/AIDS. Integrating these activities into the school timetable was left to the discretion of the schools themselves.

Another intervention strategy was the training of teachers in teaching-learning about HIV/AIDS and infusing such teaching into the regular curriculum, following the guidelines provided in the KIE handbook. How they integrate teaching is left up to teachers. For this reason, the amount of time spent on HIV/AIDS education and the way in which it was incorporated within the regular curriculum vary per school.

Management

The field team consisted of a coordinator, an assistant coordinator, and 5–15 field officers, depending on the workload at the time. In addition to organizing the activities of the field team in visiting schools, the coordinator and assistant coordinator met with educational officials to secure local support for the program. All members of the team visited schools to explain the project to school officials, obtain consent from parents, carry out the interventions, and collect data for the evaluation.

Partnerships

From its inception, the program held annual meetings with partners to discuss the progress of the project and gain input for its continuation. At the local level, district education officers continuously supported the project, facilitating entry into schools and assisting with data collection for evaluation.

Key partners in both the implementation and evaluation of this program were participating schools and teachers. Teachers made their classrooms available for activities, carried out activities, and provided a wealth of information for the evaluation. The funding partners for the project were the Partnership for Child Development and the World Bank.

Evaluation

Evaluating the impact of an HIV prevention program is especially challenging, for three main reasons:

- Sexual behavior cannot be directly observed.

- Self-reports of behavior can be untruthful and are likely to be biased by the program itself (that is, once members of the target group become aware of the behavioral prescriptions of the program, they are more likely to report the prescribed behavior than their actual behavior).

- Reductions in biological indicators of unsafe behaviors (such as childbearing or HIV incidence) are difficult to detect. Past studies of HIV/AIDS education programs have suffered from small sample sizes, which reduced their ability to measure program effectiveness and draw conclusions.

Evaluation of this program was conducted with these challenges in mind. The first step in the design of the study was to identify an outcome measure that was believable and could be collected easily. Testing students for HIV was not an option, because of budgetary reasons. Instead, the incidence of childbearing was used as a proxy outcome for unsafe sexual behavior. Care was taken to ensure that the size of the study would provide enough statistical power to detect even small changes in childbearing among teenage girls in the target group. The total number of schools needed for the study to be effective was calculated to be about 330.

Evaluation of the program was coordinated by the Poverty Action Lab at MIT. Representatives of the lab designed the project to facilitate rigorous evaluation. They coordinated collection of extensive data on a range of outcomes and carried out rigorous analysis during the course of the project, both to ensure the project's smooth running and to provide concrete information to others who could make use of the evaluation data for the development of similar HIV prevention programs.

During the course of the program, a stratified randomized evaluation was carried out in 328 schools. Randomly selected subsamples were selected to receive particular interventions. At its beginning, some 72,000 students in grades 5–8 were recruited to the study.

Teacher Training

The teacher training program had a clear impact on teaching and some impact on knowledge and attitudes. It is not clear whether it reduced the risk of HIV, however. Teacher training did not reduce childbirth, although girls enrolled in schools whose teachers were trained were more likely to be married to the fathers of their children. Whether this reflected the formation of more stable partnerships (which would reduce the risk of HIV) or partnerships with older men, who are more ready to marry (which would increase the risk of HIV), was impossible to determine.

Debating and Essay Writing

Girls in schools that took part in debating and essay writing were 9 percentage points more likely to mention condoms as a way to protect against HIV and 7 percentage points more likely to agree to the statement that if used properly, condoms can prevent HIV transmission. Boys were 4 percentage points more likely to cite abstinence as a way to protect against HIV and 5 percentage points more likely to mention condoms as a method of protection. Girls in debate/essay schools were 8 percent more likely than girls in other schools to believe that it was okay to buy food from a shopkeeper who has HIV and 12 percent more likely to say that it is okay to use a condom before marriage if one cannot abstain from sex.

These increases in knowledge did appear to have an effect on behavior; among sexually active students, boys in schools that participated in the debate and essay competition were 12 percent more like to report having ever used a condom and 18 percent more likely to report having used a condom during last intercourse. This change occurred without an increase in self-reported sexual activity.

Sugar Daddy Talk

Providing students with information on HIV rates by age and gender led to a large reduction in the number of girls engaging in unprotected cross-generational sex. Girls exposed to the information were 65 percent less likely than other girls to have started childbearing with adult partners. Self-reported sexual activity with same-age partners increased, but childbearing by teenage couples did not. Self-reported data suggest an increase in the use of condoms by both young women and young men. Overall, girls exposed to the sugar-daddy talk were about one-third less likely to bear children the following year (figure 7.1).

Free School Uniforms

Provision of free school uniforms appeared very successful in keeping students in school: students who received free uniforms were 15 percent less

Figure 7.1: Impact of Sugar-Daddy Talk on Grade 8 Girls

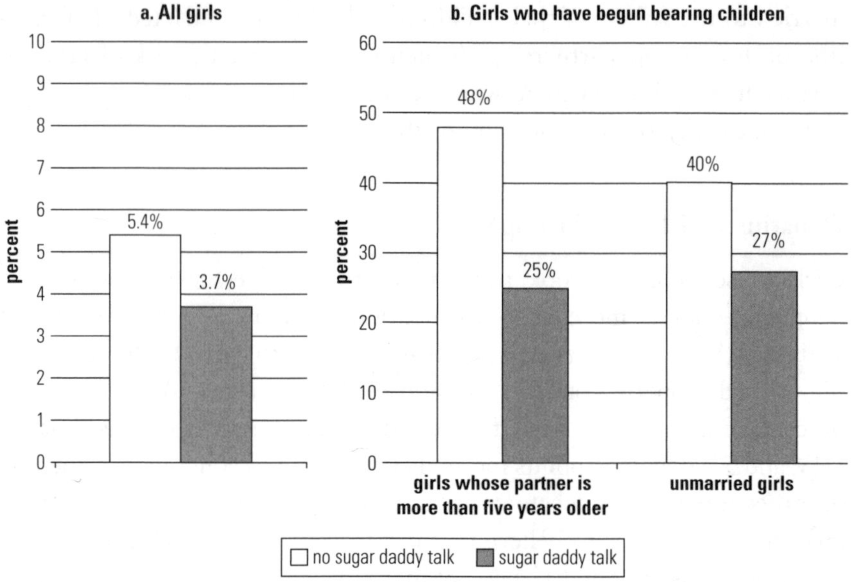

a. All girls

5.4%
3.7%

b. Girls who have begun bearing children

48%
25%

girls whose partner is
more than five years older

40%
27%

unmarried girls

□ no sugar daddy talk   ■ sugar daddy talk

Source: Primary School AIDS Prevention Program.
Note: Figure shows effect of sugar daddy talk given in the spring of 2004 on outcomes in the fall of 2005. Differences are statistically significant at the 95 percent confidence level.

likely to drop out than students who did not. Girls who received free uniforms were 10 percent less likely to have started childbearing than girls who did not. These results suggest that the program reduced the incidence of risky sexual behavior (figure 7.2).

Cost-Effectiveness

Over the program's three-year period, the teacher training component cost $67,320 ($408 per school, $146 per teacher). Assuming that only the cohort of students enrolled in grade 5 and higher at the time of the training benefited from the program, the cost per student was $2. The cost of running debating and essay writing programs in 82 schools—which reached 8,000 students—was $8,900 ($109 per school, $1.10 per student). The cost of the sugar-daddy talk—which was implemented in 71 schools, where it reached 2,500 students—was $2,000 ($28.20 per school, $0.80 per student). Based on these figures, the estimated cost per pregnancy averted was $91.

The full effect on HIV transmission of the substitution away from older partners and toward younger partners witnessed among teenage girls as a result of this program is difficult to measure with the data collected so far. Based on the HIV prevalence rates among different age groups, the data

Figure 7.2: Effects of Free School Uniforms on Grade 6 Girls

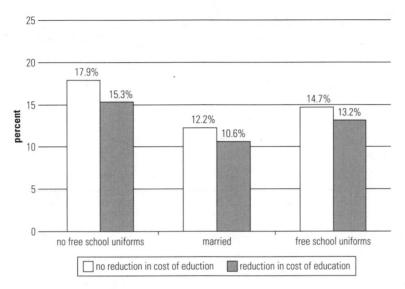

Source: Primary School AIDS Prevention Program.

Note: Figure shows effect of providing free school uniforms in the spring of 2003 on outcomes in the fall of 2005. Results are statistically significant at the 90 percent confidence level.

imply a reduction in HIV infection, but the size of this reduction is unknown. A follow-up study will be conducted in 2007–08, in which biomarkers (tests in which specific physical traits are used to measure or indicate the progress of a disease or condition) will be used.

The provision of school uniforms costs about $10.80 per male student and $12.00 per female student over the three years. The cost per pregnancy averted is estimated at $300 (table 7.2).

Lessons Learned

Several lessons can be drawn from Kenya's experience.

Measuring Impact

In many programs implementation of activities is planned first, with consideration given to monitoring and evaluation only later. Lack of early consideration of monitoring and evaluation (M&E) often makes it difficult to conduct activities that are effective, meaningful, and rigorous. Failure to take good baseline measurements at the outset, for example, makes it difficult to measure impact.

Table 7.2: Impact and Estimated Cost of Program Components

COMPONENT/DESCRIPTION	KEY EFFECTS	COST PER STUDENT	ESTIMATED COST PER PREGNANCY AVERTED
Teacher training: Trained primary-school teachers on HIV/AIDS education methodology recommended by MoEST	• Increased tolerance of people living with HIV/AIDS • Increased marriage rate among girls who started childbearing • Did not affect childbearing	$2.00	No evidence that intervention averted pregnancy
Debating and essay writing: Encouraged schools to organize student debates on condoms and essay-writing contest on ways students can protect themselves from HIV	• Increased students' knowledge • Increased likelihood of boys reporting having used condoms • Did not affect self-reported sexual activity	$1.10	—
Sugar-daddy talk: Showed video about dangers of relationships with older men (video did not mention HIV/AIDS); provided information on HIV infection rates by sex and age	• Reduced teenage childbearing with older men	$0.80	$91
Free school uniforms: Provided primary-school students with two free uniforms, thereby making school more affordable	• Reduced dropout rates • Reduced teenage childbearing and marriage	$10.80 (boys) $12.00 (girls)	$300

Source: Abdul Latif Jameel Poverty Action Lab.
— Not available.

A key aspect of the design of the Kenyan program was to ensure that the planning of impact M&E activities occurred in tandem with the planning of program implementation activities. This resulted in exceptionally high-quality monitoring and evaluation.

Implementing Culturally Acceptable Interventions

School-based HIV prevention is fraught with ideological positions and strong views about what is and is not appropriate to teach to school children. Views differ, for example, on whether it is acceptable for teachers to teach condom use.

By careful and creative thinking, the program was able to employ successful HIV prevention approaches that were both effective and culturally and politically uncontroversial. The use of debates and essay-writing competitions enabled students to engage with difficult issues without teachers being seen as taking the lead.

Sustaining Political Support

Effective HIV prevention demands long-term, sustained activities and support. Gaining and maintaining the support needed for activities to occur is often difficult, because different stakeholders place different emphasis on what programs should do. Without strong and broad-based support, programs are likely to be unsustainable and unstable.

To ensure broad acceptability of the findings and increased chances of scale up, it is very important to involve as many stakeholders as possible in program design. Key stakeholders in the Kenyan government were involved in the project from its inception, through high-level annual meetings at which progress and results were discussed. The showcasing of the results of the program in the *2007 World Development Report*: *Development and the Next Generation*, as well as articles on the program in the popular press, will make international stakeholders and policy makers aware of the program's achievement.

Conclusion

Kenya's primary-school HIV prevention program is a remarkable example of the ways in which a small number of well-designed and simple school-based interventions can have a measurable impact on factors that lead to the transmission of HIV. Documentation of the efficacy of three of the program's components—debating and essay writing, sugar-daddy talk, and provision of free school uniforms—increases their long-term sustainability as well as the likelihood that they will be scaled up across Kenya.

Annex 7.1

Primary School AIDS Prevention Attainment of Impact Benchmarks

BENCHMARK	ATTAINMENT/COMMENT
1. Identifies and focuses on specific sexual health goals	✓ Focused on reducing HIV and other STIs and decreasing pregnancies among young women.
2. Focuses narrowly on specific behaviors that lead to sexual health goals	*Debating and essay writing:* ✓ Allowed students to identify specific behaviors that can help them avoid HIV infection.
	Sugar-daddy talk: ✓ Discouraged cross-generational sex, which decreases risk of HIV infection among young people.
	Free school uniforms: ✓ Discouraged students from leaving primary school, which helps prevent early pregnancies.

(Continues on the following page)

BENCHMARK	ATTAINMENT/COMMENT
3. Identifies and focuses on sexual psychosocial risk and protective factors that are highly related to each of these behaviors	*Debating and essay writing:* ✓ Allowed students to identify risks and develop strategies for overcoming them. *Sugar-daddy talk:* ✓ Discouraged cross-generational sex. *Free school uniforms:* ✓ Discouraged students from leaving primary school.
4. Implements multiple activities to change each of the selected risk and protective factors	✓ Included lectures, debating, essay writing, videos, and discussions.
5. Actively involves youth by creating a safe social environment	*Free school uniforms:* ✓ Kept some students in school, a relatively safe social environment.
6. Employs a variety of teaching methods designed to involve participants and have them personalize the information	✓ Included lectures, debating, essay writing, videos, and discussions.
7. Conveys clear message about sexual activity and condom or contraceptive use and continually reinforces that message	*Debating and essay writing:* Partial. Gave students opportunity to think critically about contraceptives.
8. Includes effective curricula and activities appropriate to the age, sexual experience, and culture of participating students	*Debating and essay writing:* ✓ Gave students opportunity to engage individually with the material, ensuring that their own experiences inform their activity.
9. Increases knowledge by providing basic, accurate information about the risks of teen sexual activity and methods of avoiding intercourse or using protection against pregnancy and STIs	*Debating and essay writing:* ✓ Built on information that some students already had to strengthen their understanding and spread information to peers. *Sugar-daddy talk:* ✓ Provided information about a specific risk of teenage sexual activity.
10. Uses some of the same strategies to change perceptions of peer values, to recognize peer pressure to have sex, and to address that pressure	*Sugar-daddy talk:* Partial. Discouraged cross-generational sex, which is common in the region.
11. Identifies specific situations that might lead to sex, unwanted sex, or unprotected sex and identifies methods of avoiding those situations or getting out of them	*Sugar-daddy talk:* ✓ Identified presence of sugar daddies and showed video in which characters avoid cross-generational sex to protect themselves from HIV.
12. Provides modeling of and practice with communication, negotiation, and refusal skills to improve both skills and self-efficacy in using those skills	*Debating and essay writing:* Partial. Gave students chance to articulate ways of preventing HIV through speaking and writing.

Source: Authors.

Annex 7.2

Contact Information

International Child Support
PO Box 599
Busia, Kenya
Contact person: Grace Makana, HIV Education Project Coordinator
Phone: +254 (0) 722

Abdul Latif Jameel Poverty Action Lab
Massachusetts Institute of Technology
E52-243B
50 Memorial Drive
Cambridge, MA 02142-1347
povertyactionlab@mit.edu
Contact person: Rachel Glennerster, Executive Director
Phone: +1-617-324-0108

Available materials
Two detailed reports are available at http://www.povertyactionlab.com/
projects/project.php?pid=5. The reports, as well as copies of the questionnaires used for the evaluation, can be obtained from Pascaline Dupas
(pascaline.dupas@gmail.com).

References

Gallant, M., and E. Maticka-Tyndale. 2004. "School-Based HIV Prevention Programmes for African Youth." *Social Science & Medicine* 58 (7): 1337–51.

Government of Kenya. 2003. *Demographic and Health Survey*. Nairobi.

Ministry of Health. 2001. *AIDS in Kenya*. Nairobi.

UNICEF (United Nations Children's Fund). 2006. *The State of the World's Children*.
New York: UNICEF.

Window of Hope at a Glance

Description: School-based extracurricular HIV/AIDS and life-skills education

Number of participating schools: Teachers in 1,055 public primary schools (85 percent) have been trained in the junior (grades 4 and 5) modules and 787 (64 percent) in the senior (grades 6 and 7) modules.

Coverage: 17,930 students in 37 percent of the country's public primary schools in all 13 regions of the country

Target groups: School-going children 9–14 in government primary schools. Secondary target audience includes upper-primary school teachers, parents and guardians, and the wider community.

Components: After-school clubs. Eventually, HIV/AIDS education will be integrated into two carrier subjects.

Establishment and duration: Begun in 2003, envisaged as ongoing program

Management: Managed and implemented by the HIV/AIDS Management Unit (HAMU) of the Ministry of Basic Education, Sport and Culture (MBESC), with technical assistance from UNICEF

Role of HAMU: HAMU coordinates, manages, and implements the program.

Role of key partners: UNICEF provides technical assistance.

Cost: About $275,000 a year ($30 per student)

Key evaluation results: A needs assessment revealed the following findings:

- Students in upper-primary school are more concerned about getting the "big picture" than learning specific details about HIV/AIDS and sex.

- The majority of teachers recognize the need for HIV education in the school curriculum and feel that it is their obligation to do what they can to help their learners stay healthy. A minority of teachers is not willing to talk about sex and teach skills such as condom use.

- Teachers have a wide variety of training needs, from teaching methods to counseling skills to specific questions about topics related to sexual health.

- Many teachers report needing more materials and resources effectively to teach sexual health and HIV prevention.

CHAPTER 8

The Window of Hope Program, Namibia

Transmission of HIV is increasingly understood to occur as the result of a complex interplay of factors, including individual decision making, societal forces, cultural attitudes, and environmental determinants. If school-age children are to learn how to grow up able to remain free of HIV, merely equipping them with information about the virus is not enough. To be effective, education must also address issues of life skills, motivation, and the environment.

Namibia's Window of Hope program is an example of an attempt to develop such a comprehensive response. Delivered through after-school clubs, the program aims to equip 9- to 14-year-olds with self-esteem, knowledge, attitudes, and skills before they become sexually active and risk behaviors become ingrained.

> This is a program that was developed by Namibians, within Namibia, based on some impor-
> tant Namibian values, taking culture into consideration, so it's not something strange. It is not
> only about jumping and screaming to children about HIV/AIDS and its effects, but is also a
> program that is life-skills based, to help children learn skills that are critical in surviving
> among the current waves of the epidemic.
>
> *Program Implementer*

A major challenge facing those responsible for HIV/AIDS education is curriculum reform. How can the school curriculum be strengthened to include accurate age-appropriate information on HIV/AIDS to support acquisition of essential knowledge and life skills? How can educators best

Shamani Jeffrey Shikwambi and Alicia Fentiman, consultants, conducted the interviews and collected the data for this chapter. Silke Felton and Rushnan Murtaza, UNICEF, Namibia; Lucy Steinitz, Ministry of Education, Namibia; and Criana Connal, consultant, assisted in drafting the text of this chapter.

ensure that sexual health and HIV/AIDS education engenders positive values, attitudes, and behaviors?

Description

Rationale and History

In 2003 Namibia established a policy framework that was conducive to curricular reform. The framework demanded "age- and ability-appropriate education on HIV/AIDS . . . in the curriculum of all learners" (MBESC/MHETTEC 2003).

At the time the framework was adopted, the school curriculum did not offer a self-standing, compulsory life-skills subject. Life-skills training was allocated only one lesson a week in the school timetable. Moreover, lessons were often not taught, because teachers were assigned to the subject in a random manner.

In 2003 Namibia developed the Window of Hope program, a comprehensive life-skills education that adds an HIV education component to the existing formal curriculum and supports after-school clubs (figure 8.1). The program is managed and implemented by the HIV/AIDS Management Unit (HAMU) of the Ministry of Basic Education, Sport and Culture (MBESC), with technical assistance from UNICEF. Targeting the crucial "window of opportunity" in adolescent behavior formation, the program equips 9- to 14-year-olds with self-esteem, knowledge, attitudes, and skills before they become sexually active and risk behaviors become ingrained.

Following an audit of all subject curricula in senior-primary school and a nationwide study of the status of HIV/AIDS education, a national workshop was held. During the workshop, stakeholders agreed on an integration framework in which two examinable subjects—natural science and health education and social studies—were identified as the core carrier subjects for

Figure 8.1: Timeline of Window of Hope Implementation

2003	2004	2005
National study on needs of upper-primary teachers and learners conducted; two national stakeholders' workshops held; program designed.	Junior modules finalized. Thirty-two education officers from 13 regional directorates trained as Window of Hope trainers; 655 teachers from 572 schools trained. Eight of 13 regions achieved more than 80 percent coverage of all primary schools.	Senior modules finalized; Window of Hope trainers trained on senior modules; teacher training on junior and senior modules rolled out.

Source: Authors.

HIV-related skills. Having endorsed this framework the ministry's responsible decision-making body on curriculum reform revised the syllabi of the two carrier subjects.

As of 2007 the program's in-school component had not yet been implemented. Accordingly, this chapter focuses on the extracurricular component, which was based on lessons learned from the *My Future My Choice* intervention (an earlier life-skills program implemented in Namibia) and on recommendations of the national study conducted to develop an in-school program component. The design process was singular in its emphasis on participatory and culturally sensitive design, including active collaboration with a range of national stakeholders as well as school children in rural and urban areas, parents, and representatives of religious organizations.

Program design reflected several factors:

- The need to reach children at an early age, when their behavior can still be shaped and most are enrolled in school.

- The need for a holistic approach, combining both knowledge and skills for prevention and the building of psychosocial coping mechanisms in a society that has been profoundly affected by HIV/AIDS. Such an approach also seeks the best way to address inequalities between boys and girls, making sure that girls are equally empowered.

- The importance of long-term commitment to children's well-being. The program consists of not just a few concise sessions but a series of meetings over a period of up to four years. The program also stresses the active involvement of parents and guardians in the after-school clubs, as facilitators or facilitators' assistants, to create deeper communication channels between parents and children.

- The challenge of developing a program that is suitable for Namibia's culturally, linguistically, and ethnically diverse population.

The importance of delivering the messages early enough

In Namibia, people are realizing now that in light of the current programs that are targeting adolescents and young adults as far as their sexuality is concerned, something was missing. That missing puzzle is the fact that children are being reached very late with sexuality-related messages that may be able to influence their attitudes and behaviors. The government recognized the need for children to receive information much more early on in life. Thus, in wanting to change behavior, it was realized it was better to target children when they are still young rather than when they are already in the adolescence period and may be engaging in some risky behaviors already.

Program Implementer

The significance of providing accurate and relevant information

Because it is hard for some people to see HIV/AIDS in their own back yards, it is important to provide information. Not any type of information but the correct information supported by research. Once they have the information, the next step is empowerment . . . the self-confidence to be able to stick to their own decisions. The ability to survive peer pressure is critical for many children and young people, in light of the current HIV/AIDS crisis in Namibia. . . . HIV/AIDS is ruining the fabric of life, there is need to give children hope in the midst of this catastrophe. That is why such an aim of empowering children and giving them hope to live through all the midst of all the death going on in the country is important, I believe.

Program Implementer

The program design was finalized and tested in both urban and rural areas, under the supervision of two MBESC–led steering groups. The program was launched in 2004, during AIDS Awareness Week, when after-school Window of Hope clubs were declared an official extracurricular activity by MBESC. In 2005 training in the program was extended to nongovernmental organizations (NGOs), community-based organizations (CBOs), and some faith-based organizations (FBOs). Little or no data on these organizations' activities are available, however.

Planned activities for the future include ensuring that trained schools use the monitoring and reporting system, which is designed to tie in with routine reporting structures at the circuit (local), regional, and national level.

Aims, Objectives, and Strategies

The aim of the program is to build resilience and develop self-esteem in upper-primary school learners so that they can become strong and healthy adults who will be able to face the challenges of society, including HIV/AIDS; to prepare learners to care for others and to deal with illness and death; and to help them combat the stigmatization associated with HIV/AIDS.

The program objectives are to:

• equip participants with relevant knowledge and information

• build skills for decision making, and learning to say no to peers and adults

• develop self-esteem and self-confidence in participants

• promote participants' personal decision making with respect to sexual behavior

• encourage participants to take concrete steps to envisage and realize a future

- develop in participants a sense of self and a sense of others

- encourage participants to adopt an attitude of care and cooperation

- cope with the death of a family member

- deal with the stigma and discrimination associated with HIV/AIDS.

The program uses several strategies to impart information on HIV prevention, empower learners, promote healthy sexual behavior, and teach communication-skills learners. These strategies include:

- empowering participants with behavior-change information

- engaging participants in story-telling sessions that teach them that they are strong and clever

- having participants think about their aspirations in life and take steps to work toward achieving those aspirations

- engaging participants in cooperative activities

- teaching participants to share and respect one another

- helping participants learn to be compassionate toward others.

Target Groups

The program targets all Namibian children aged 9–14. The program was originally restricted to children enrolled in school; it is now open to all children aged 9–14, whether or not they are enrolled in school. A secondary target group is upper-primary school teachers, parents and guardians, and the wider community.

Components

The after-school clubs follow a teacher-led club model. Activities include sharing of information, thoughts, and feelings; games, songs, drama, art, and music; visualization exercises, story-telling, acting-out sessions, and sharing sessions to promote a sense of openness; lectures; and visits to clinics and interactions with people living with HIV.

Up to 30 children form a junior club (for grade 4 and 5 students) or a senior club (for grade 6 and 7 students). If more than 30 children are interested in joining, more than one club is formed. Membership is voluntary. The clubs meet once a week, immediately after school, in a designated classroom or place in the school grounds, for about 90 minutes. Children usually participate in the clubs for four years.

Box 8.1: Typical Opening Ritual

Children hold lighted candles and form a circle around the Window of Hope flag. They then engage in a particular ritual, depending on the stage of the program. One ritual used is the thundercloud ritual. It goes like this:

Words spoken	Movement made
Feel it proud	Pull out your chest and hold up your fists.
Say out loud	Raise your voice and cup your hands around your mouth.
We are the green sound	Rub your hands in circles together to make a swishing sound.
Window of Hope	Patter your feet, like the sound of rain.
Thundercloud!	Shout out the word, then clap your hands once.

Sessions begin with a ritual, which is repeated regularly in more or less the same way. This ritual gives the session a structure and rhythm, and it creates a sense of belonging and security for the children (box 8.1).

Teachers and facilitators are encouraged to ensure that clubs include a balance of girls and boys; children who are affected by HIV/AIDS, including orphans; children who have problems in class, such as poor concentration and lack of self-esteem; and children who live in hostels (orphans or children separated from their families for various reasons).

Club sessions are divided into eight self-contained modules, called "windows," each with its own color, theme, and activities. Each window consists of five compulsory sessions of 90 minutes each. If clubs meet once a week, the time required for completion of a window is five weeks.

Implementation

The Window of Hope is a national program implemented across Namibia (table 8.1). During the program's first two years, it trained 1,341 teachers from 1,055 schools in the junior modules and 983 teachers from 787 schools in the senior modules. As of October 2006, 85 percent of public primary schools had teachers trained in the junior windows and 64 percent had teachers trained in the senior windows.

Staff Selection and Training

Window of Hope trainers are selected by the regional director of education, based on their ability to work with children and to discuss sexuality without inhibition. Trainers are trained during a four- to five-day workshop that takes place in Windhoek (Namibia's capital) or in a regional capital.

Table 8.1: Coverage of Window of Hope Program, 2006*

REGION	NUMBER OF TEACHERS TRAINED		NUMBER OF SCHOOLS COMPLETING ONE WINDOW	NUMBER OF SCHOOLS COMPLETING TWO WINDOWS	NUMBER OF LEARNERS COMPLETING AT LEAST FOUR SESSIONS	
	JUNIOR MODULES	SENIOR MODULES			BOYS	GIRLS
Caprivi	88	63	0	32	610	842
Erongo	49	46	21	4	781	916
Hardap	45	47	11	29	844	1160
Karas	48	48	12	16	483	835
Kavango	203	155	46	96	1,711	1,744
Khomas	73	23	7	4	116	228
Kunene	46	46	24	10	509	808
Ohangwena	204	91	46	8	707	1,079
Omaheke	29	51	0	13	593	832
Omusati	220	55	21	6	422	601
Oshana	107	66	28	14	498	827
Oshikoto	172	86	7	8	314	470
Total	1,284	777	223	240	7,588	10,342

Source: HIV and AIDS Management Unit.

* This table gives data for 12 of Namibia's regions. Otjozondjupa is not included.

The training is provided by program consultants and senior-school counselors from MBESC.

Teachers participating in the program are selected by their schools (figure 8.2). They must teach grade 4–7, exhibit an interest in the program, and commit to facilitating the program during after-schools hours. Teacher trainees participate in a four- to five-day workshop, at which they are trained by regional trainers. A five-day training curriculum was also developed that equips teachers and NGO workers to facilitate both junior and senior modules. Training stresses the importance of involving parents, caregivers, and guardians in program activities.

Training methods include lectures; role-playing; acting-out sessions; storytelling; drawing; working in groups, pairs, and individually; reading assignments; and open discussion formats. One-day refresher training is

---

On the importance of including parents/caregivers/guardians in Window of Hope activities

. . . it needs to be done in conjunction with parenting. Everything we are teaching children at school, it is ideal that parents at home reinforce that. After all, parents are the first teachers of their children . . . but we also realize that when it comes to issues relating to sexuality no one wants to talk about it, even parents. That leaves as us teachers to do the work. As educators we have a moral obligation towards children to give them all the necessary tools for future survival. I guess that is our job.

Training Facilitator

Figure 8.2: Forming a Window of Hope Club

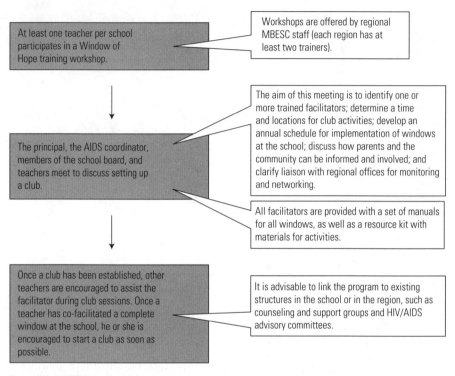

Source: HIV and AIDS Management Unit.

offered that provides an opportunity to measure progress in program implementation, address challenges and obstacles that may have arisen during implementation, and reinforce personal motivation for participating in the program.

On the importance of equipping teachers/facilitators with the necessary knowledge and skills

It all depends on your own comfort level about sexuality. If you have not been informed yourself and you are not comfortable talking about issues of sexuality, it is hard to do so. The best is to detach your own emotions and values, and wear your teacher's hat proudly and do the work. I don't necessarily agree with everything I teach, or enjoy it, but I also know it is not about me but the learners. So I got to give it all I got and what I got is my best for now.

Program Implementer

Field support is provided in the following ways:

• Regional resource centers provide access to information on HIV/AIDS.

• Cluster meetings allow facilitators, trainers, and HIV/AIDS coordinators to exchange views and experiences and develop networks.

- Inspectors, advisory teachers, HIV/AIDS coordinators, and Window of Hope trainers visit schools to assess the clubs. The school principal periodically attends sessions, monitoring the quality of activities. The School Board includes the Window of Hope program as part of its supervisory responsibilities.

- Meetings with parents and guardians are held during which they are informed about Window of Hope activities and given the opportunity to voice and seek responses to concerns.

Materials

A key feature of the materials design process, which took place over an 18-month period, was its inclusion of inputs from educators, nurses, community leaders, traditional healers, and parents, as well as, HAMU, UNICEF, and two Namibian consultants. The materials underwent a lengthy testing process that solicited feedback from children 9–14. A set of materials was developed for use by both trainers and teachers/facilitators. The *Junior Window of Hope Manual* is for grades 4 and 5; the *Senior Window of Hope Manual* is for grades 6 and 7. Each manual is made up of four windows (table 8.2). Two other manuals were developed for teacher training. A parent-targeted manual, *Let's Talk with Our Children*, was also developed.

Each window includes five 90-minute sessions of participatory activities (table 8.3). Instructions for each session are spelled out in detail in the manuals, which also provide background information on the developmental stages of adolescents and the themes dealt with in the sessions, such as self-esteem, decision making, child abuse, gender roles, reproductive health, and HIV/AIDS. Each module also provides suggestions for open, child-led activities.

In addition to the manuals, guidelines for preparing and conducting a five-day workshop were prepared (*Training Manual for Junior Windows/Senior Windows*). A CD with music to accompany all the songs in the manuals was also produced as a training and teaching aid.

Schools participating in the Window of Hope program are also equipped with a resource kit containing materials for activities such as flip-charts (illustrated teaching aids), a flag, attendance sheets, evaluation forms, and certificates and badges, given to participants on completion of each window.

Monitoring

A monitoring system for ongoing assessment of the program has been designed but has not yet been made operational. The system includes an attendance sheet completed by a facilitator following each club session and an evaluation form on completion of each window/module. The evaluation form

Table 8.2: Objectives and Topics of Program Windows

WINDOW	NAME	OBJECTIVES	TOPICS
Junior windows			
Green	We Window	• Develop self-awareness and self-esteem among participants. • Help participants learn to express and share good and bad feelings. • Encourage participants to help others in times of distress.	• I am a special person • Expressing and sharing feelings • Helping each other to feel better
Yellow	Window of Change	• Help participants develop positive attitudes toward their changing bodies and feeling. • Help participants deal with their physical and emotional changes. • Help participants develop understanding and respect for the opposite sex.	• My changing body • Can boys and girls be friends? • Understanding and respecting the opposite sex
Blue	Yes and No Window	• Teach participants to say yes to things that are good for them. • Teach participants to say no to things that are bad for them and their future.	• Good touch and bad touch • I am the boss of my body • Learning to say no, learning to say yes • Making decisions as a group
Red	Power Window	• Teach participants how to protect against HIV. • Help participants fight stigmatization. • Encourage participants to help people living with AIDS.	• We are clever (we know what HIV/AIDS is) • We are strong (we can protect ourselves against HIV/AIDS) • We accept people with HIV/AIDS (we care for people)
Senior windows			
Purple	I–We Window	• Develop self-esteem and self-awareness in each participant. • Develop a sense of belonging to different groups. • Develop team spirit and encourage a culture of caring for one another.	• I am special, you are special, we are special • Good friends are important • We are all part of a family
Lime	Window of Love	• Help participants understand and deal with love, sex, and sexuality, so that they can make responsible and healthy decisions.	• The gifts and risks of sexuality • Equality between boys and girls • Different forms of love
Turquoise	Double Yes/ Double No Window	• Help participants learn assertiveness skills. • Help participants make positive and sustainable decisions. • Help participants transform decisions into actions.	• The steps toward my future • Making decisions • Learning to say no
Orange	Double-Power Window	• Equip children with knowledge about HIV/AIDS. • Empower them, through knowledge and self-confidence, to protect themselves against HIV. • Encourage attitudes of responsibility and caring for people who have lost loved ones to illness and for those who are ill.	• Right and wrong ideas about HIV/AIDS • Protecting ourselves against HIV • Testing, treatment, and emotional care

Source: HIV and AIDS Management Unit.

Table 8.3: Opening Rituals and Activities for the Red Window

COMPONENT	OPENING RITUAL	ACTIVITIES
Session 1: We Are Clever	Getting to know one another	• Sharing: We Have to Be Clever! • Quiz: What Is True and False about AIDS? • Game: The Newspaper Game • Song: H-I Virus, We Beat You • Puppet show: The H-I Virus Puppet Show
Session 2: We Are Strong	Attack on the human body	• Puppet show: The H-I Virus Puppet Show • Song: The Power Song • Art: My Star
Session 3: We Accept People	Why children are stigmatized	• Game: The Stigmatization Game • Acting: Maria's Mother • Story: Visiting Mr. Hausiku
Session 4: We Care for People Who Are Sick	What can we do for sick people?	• Song: Kumbaya, My Lord • Game: The Ambulance Game • Art: Get-Well Card • Story: The Wooden Bowl
Session 5: Review	Looking back	• Singing and games • Art: Red ribbon poster • Closing ceremony: Certificates and badges
Suggestions for additional sessions		
Glossary		
Annex: Helping Children Deal with Grief and Death		

Source: HIV and AIDS Management Unit.

solicits information about the number of children completing a window and the impact in terms of acquisition of new information, development of communication skills, ability to participate in a group, changes in self-confidence and attitudes, enjoyment during participation, and behavior during sessions; the school principal will forward the evaluation forms to the circuit inspector, who will compile a circuit-level summary form, which will be submitted to Window of Hope trainers or the HIV/AIDS coordinator at regional level. A focal point will compile a regional summary form, which will be submitted to HAMU, the body responsible for producing and distributing a national program summary report.

Advocacy

Given its bold aims and innovative methods, the importance of advocacy in a program such as Window of Hope cannot be overstated. Advocacy efforts entailed the inclusion of parents in the design process and the introduction of a parent-targeted manual, *Let's Talk with Our Children*. Support from religious bodies was generated through their participation in both program design and training activities, with some churches offering to use Window of Hope materials as part of their Sunday school curriculum. Ongoing advocacy methods include regional education officers' meetings; orientation meetings for government officials, such as school inspectors, regional governors, and advisory officers; and continuous consultation between HAMU and UNICEF. Both project managers and implementers stress the need continually to use these and other conventional methods (national TV, leaflets) of advocacy to stimulate support for the program.

Cost

The program cost about $250,000–$300,000 a year during 2004–05 ($27.80–$33.35 per learner). The main budget lines were program development (writing and testing of manuals and activities), teacher training, and training supplies.

Evaluation

No evaluation of program activities or impact has been undertaken. However, the design of the program was based on a national study undertaken in October 2003 by MBESC, as part of the education sector's strategic plan to strengthen sexual health and HIV/AIDS education across the basic education curriculum. This research focused primarily on the upper-primary phase of school (grades 5–7), which forms the heart of sexual health education in the Namibian curriculum.

Five questions guided the research:

- What health issues affect learners and their communities?

- What, if anything, do learners want and need to learn about sexual health and HIV/AIDS to maintain their sexual health?

- Are teachers prepared to deliver sexual health and HIV/AIDS education in the classroom comfortably and effectively?

- What are teachers' training needs regarding sexual health and HIV/AIDS education?

- What resources and materials do teachers need to effectively teach sexual health and HIV/AIDS education?

Methodology

Forty-five schools in Caprivi, Erongo, Karas, Kavango, Kunene, Ohangwena, Omaheke, Omusati, Oshana, Oshikoto, Otjiwarango, Rehoboth, Tsumeb, and Windhoek (urban and rural) participated in the study. Some 211 teachers of natural science and health education, life skills/guidance, and social studies (62 percent of them women) and 528 learners from grades 6 and 7 participated in the study.

Eighteen National Institute for Educational Development (NIED) officials, mostly curriculum developers, and two regional education officers worked together on 11 data-collection teams. Data-collection methods included self-assessment tools for teachers and for schools, focus group discussions, and learners' drawing exercises.

Key Findings

Assessment of the program yielded several key findings.

Learners' needs

Namibian students need and want comprehensive sexual health and HIV/AIDS education to prepare them to lead sexually healthy lives and manage the impact HIV/AIDS is having on them. The most commonly asked questions concerned where HIV comes from, how it got to Namibia, when the epidemic will end, and when a cure will be found.

Teachers identified learner needs regarding managing the impact of HIV/AIDS (caring for sick people, living positively, coping). They also identified learners' need to understand condom use and how to say no to sex.

Learners need specific skills, such as communication, negotiation, self-awareness, analyzing, decision making, and problem solving. Situations identified by teachers and learners include pressure to have sex, pressure not to use condoms, the influence of money on sexual relationships, sexual advances from adults, substance abuse, and power imbalances between males and females in sexual relationships.

The majority of teachers recognized the need for HIV/AIDS education in the school curriculum and felt an obligation to do what they can to help their learners stay healthy. A small minority of teachers was not willing to talk about sex or to teach skills such as condom use.

Training needs of teachers

Ninety-six percent of teachers report that they felt confident about their basic knowledge about sexual health and HIV/AIDS. Most (89 percent) reported that they felt comfortable talking about sexual health issues with students. Forty-three percent indicated that they needed in-service training on at least one aspect of teaching about sexual health, such as teaching methods, sensitivity to different cultures in class, approaching shy or negative students, and teaching in mixed-gender peer groups.

Teachers have a wide variety of training needs, from teaching methods to counseling skills to specific questions about sexual health–related topics. The training needs most frequently cited by teachers were guidance and counseling skills, home-based care, teaching methods/skills, overall training, and proper use of condoms. Teachers need training on general life skills (interpreting, analyzing, and synthesizing information; problem solving; making informed choices; and building self-esteem). They also need training on the relation between abstinence and safe sex education. Many teachers feel that the messages of abstinence and safe sex are mutually exclusive rather than complementary.

Materials needed by teachers

Although teachers and learners reported that they have access to a broad range of materials and resources on HIV/AIDS—posters, TV and radio programs, textbooks, brochures and pamphlets, newspapers—many reported that they need more materials and resources to be effective. The most pressing need is for visual materials, particularly videos that show people living with HIV/AIDS, so that learners "believe the disease is real." Some teachers reported that they need condoms, so that they can demonstrate how to use them. Some teachers also requested that textbooks be revised to reflect more sexual health and HIV/AIDS education.

Lessons Learned

Schools in Namibia have demonstrated a high level of interest in the Window of Hope program. Interviews with program managers and implementers reveal several of the challenges they face and some solutions to them.

Lack of Trained Teachers

Too few teachers have been trained to facilitate Window of Hope clubs (and eventually to provide in-class lessons). The lack of available teachers and trainers is in part a result of the exodus of teachers from the profession. Transfer of teachers also disrupts the program.

The number of teachers needs to increase and the scope of training sessions broadened. When the program is made part of the formal curriculum, training will become part of preservice teacher education at teacher training colleges across the country. A module for teacher training institutions that incorporates both Windows of Hope and *My Future Is My Choice* is being prepared.

The program stresses the importance of including community members and parents, guardians, and caregivers as facilitators. This strategy could be promoted as a partial solution to the lack of trained teachers. In the words of one program facilitator, "It would be great to see a teacher and a parent work together in every club around the country." Program planners also envisage the training of older children as program facilitators.

Teaching Motivation

Participation in the program increases the burden on teachers. As one program facilitator noted, "There is a constant influx of information about HIV/AIDS being sent to educators, which takes up a lot of their time. They are near to burn-out about HIV/AIDS." Lack of interest in or commitment to the program on the part of the school administration or community can make this burden particularly difficult to bear.

Ensuring that teachers' motivation to participate in the program is not undermined involves a combination of responses. First, the school administration could ensure that teachers who facilitate Window of Hope clubs are excused from other extracurricular responsibilities. Second, school authorities and administration could prioritize certain HIV/AIDS–related interventions, allowing teachers to maximize their time and capacities. The prioritizing of the Window of Hope program would be in keeping with MBESC's decision to roll out the program as the country's official extracurricular HIV/AIDS education-related initiative. Third, advocacy efforts could be intensified, aiming to generate and strengthen support from education authorities and ensuring local communities' sense of ownership and commitment to the program.

Language

Program implementers and facilitators have expressed concerns about the program's language of instruction. Although English is not the first language of many children participating in the program, all manuals and supplementary materials are in English. Teachers are encouraged to translate materials into local languages where necessary and are given guidance on how to do so effectively.

The *Teachers Manual Implementation Guidelines* explicitly states the flexible and creative nature of a teacher/facilitator's role in the program:

Sometimes, you may decide to explain stories and other things in the manuals in your own words, or translate them into the children's home language, so that the material is more easily understood. That is fine. In the WINDOW OF HOPE, children should also be allowed to express themselves in whatever language they feel most comfortable in. But if you do this, it will be especially important for you to go over everything before each session. For example, if you decide to translate the stories in the local language, or tell them in your own words, you will need to practice first

Taken from the Teachers Manual Implementation Guidelines (MBESC/HAMU, 2004)

Information Sharing

A variety of ministries in Namibia provide HIV/AIDS–related interventions. These include MBESC; the Ministry of Health and Social Services; the Ministry of Gender Equity and Child Welfare; and the ministries of agriculture, water, forestry, trade and industry, and home affairs. NGOs, CBOs, FBOs, and the private sector also play a role in HIV prevention. Without multisectoral and public-private collaboration and coordination, information flows are lacking or compromised. Without the relevant data, the scope for collaboration and coordination between stakeholders is undermined. To respond to these needs, MBESC formed its HIV and AIDs Management Unit (HAMU), whose aim is to provide "a systemic and coordinated planning and management response to HIV/AIDS through improved practice and resource utilization, partnerships, and the creation of a dedicated HIV/AIDS management unit with the power and vision to guide education through the crisis" (National Strategic Plan on HIV and AIDS, 2004–2009).

On setting up a similar program within alternative cultural contexts

Take cultural values, attitudes, problems of the learners and trainers into account. Develop the program with a working group in which parents, teachers, school counselors, NGOs, church-based organizations, and so forth are represented. Their contribution creates a sense of ownership. Rolling out is possible because all stakeholders were involved in the design. . . . Once you embark to set up a program, stay the course. Don't start today and stop tomorrow; otherwise it gives the community an opportunity to again downplay the importance of HIV prevention programs.

Program Managers and Implementers

Conclusion

In the absence of a stand-alone life skills subject that is compulsory for all learners, the Window of Hope program is a step in the right direction. While advocacy continues with regard to the curricular component, the after-school component provides value in supplementing subject teaching on HIV/AIDS. It is culturally specific and student centered; it uses a participatory and playful learning style; and it emphasizes attitudes and skills that are not easily examinable, such as self-esteem, which are difficult to teach in the classroom.

It may be too early to say [what the role of a child/youth may be in terms of HIV prevention] because we will need to do some form of assessments, years down the road. But what is happening is that these children are being taught and I want to believe they are taking responsibility for their own future. They are being taught to be able to say "Yes and No" loud and clear. They are being taught to stand up for themselves, and also to stand up for others in their communities.

Program Implementer

Annex 8.1

Window of Hope Attainment of Impact Benchmarks

BENCHMARK	ATTAINMENT/COMMENT
1. Identifies and focuses on specific sexual health goals	✓ Program focuses on prevention and transmission of HIV and encourages learners to take charge of their sexual lives.
2. Focuses narrowly on specific behaviors that lead to sexual health goals	✓ Program promotes abstinence and condom use.
3. Identifies and focuses on sexual psychosocial risk and protective factors that are highly related to each of these behaviors	✓ Program generates and strengthens psychosocial protective attitudes. Skills and behaviors are fundamental aims of the program.
4. Implements multiple activities to change each of the selected risk and protective factors	✓ Program combines teacher-led and child-led activities.
5. Actively involves youth by creating a safe social environment	✓ Careful program design ensures a culturally sensitive and age-appropriate approach.
6. Employs a variety of teaching methods designed to involve participants and have them personalize the information	✓ Program uses wide range of participatory teaching methodologies.
7. Conveys a clear message about sexual activity and condom or contraceptive use and continually reinforces that message	✓ Program promotes abstinence and condom use, as well as clear messages regarding right and ability to say no.
8. Includes effective curricula and activities appropriate to the age, sexual experience, and culture of participating learners	✓ Extracurricular activities were designed in collaboration with the target age group.
9. Increases knowledge by providing basic, accurate information about the risks of teen sexual activity and methods of avoiding intercourse or using protection against pregnancy and STIs	✓ Facts about prevention and transmission are combined with information on how to live with HIV.
10. Uses some of the same strategies to change perceptions of peer values, to recognize peer pressure to have sex, and to address that pressure	✓ Although peer education is not a part of the program, vulnerability to peer pressure is recognized and addressed and communication among peers promoted.
11. Identifies specific situations that might lead to sex, unwanted sex, or unprotected sex and identifies methods of avoiding those situations or getting out of them	✓ Role-play, storytelling, acting-out sessions, and songs are used to identify and cope with situations that might lead to sex.
12. Provides modeling of and practice with communication, negotiation, and refusal skills to improve both skills and self-efficacy in using those skills	✓ Program stresses importance of learning and practicing negotiation and refusal skills.

Source: Authors.

Annex 8.2

Contact Information

Ministry of Basic Education, Sport and Culture,
HIV and AIDS Management Unit (HAMU)
Private Bag 13186
Windhoek, Namibia
Tel: +264-61-270 6125

UNICEF Namibia
P.O. Box 1706
Windhoek, Namibia
Tel: +264-61-204 6261/6111
Fax: +264-61-204 6206

Windows of Hope materials can be downloaded at http://www.hamu-nam.net/.

Reference

MBESC/MHETTEC (Ministry of Basic Education, Sport and Culture/Ministry of Higher Education) 2003. "Policy on HIV/AIDS for the Education Sector." Windhoek.

Expanded Life Planning Education (ELPE) at a Glance

Description: School-based curricular and co-curricular HIV/AIDS and life-skills education

Number of schools participating: 131 of the 324 public secondary schools in Oyo State, covering more than 425,000 students

Coverage: About 40 percent of secondary schools in Oyo State, in all 33 local government areas. Program has been replicated in the states of Bauchi, Borno Gombe, Kebbi, and Yobe.

Target groups: Students aged 9–20 of both genders and all tribes. Secondary target audience includes out-of-school youth, users of youth-friendly clinics, teachers, parents, and policy makers.

Components: Program has eight components: formal HIV/AIDS education; peer education; life-planning education/HIV prevention clubs; youth-friendly health clinics; advocacy and awareness raising; teacher training; material development and distribution; and research, monitoring, and evaluation.

Establishment: Begun in Ibadan in 1994; expanded activities to 131 public secondary schools in 1999.

Management: Team composed of four key stakeholders—the Ministry of Education, Science, and Technology (MoEST); the Ministry of Health; the Association for Reproductive and Family Health (ARFH); and the Teaching Service Commission (TESCOM)—each of which has a specific role.

Role of MoEST: Reviewing policy; legalizing and regularizing the integration of life-planning education into the school curriculum; and strengthening the ministry's approach to the new challenge. Project coordinating unit has responsibilities for other operational issues, including maintaining links with schools; conducting supervision and monitoring; liaising with other partners; distributing materials to schools; collecting data from schools; providing technical assistance to teachers; and setting standards and ensuring compliance.

Role of key partners: Overall responsibility for the project lies with ARFH, whose executive director is ELPE's project coordinator and chief accounting officer. The Ministry of Health is responsible for facilitating the integration of youth-friendly services into primary health care. As the program moves from being an innovative project to part of the day-to-day work of MoEST, the Ministry of Health is called upon to provide ongoing support and advice to the educational activities of schools at the local level. TESCOM is responsible for hiring and transferring teachers. DFID provided funding for the program through 2003.

Costs: Total expenditures totaled $767,000 during 1999–2003, about $1.78 per person.

Evaluation results: Evaluation revealed the following results:

- Peer education was effective in empowering young people in public speaking; interpersonal communication; and decision-making, problem-solving, and leadership skills. It also helped improve young people's health-seeking behavior.

- Students were able to discuss their reproductive health problems with teachers and health care providers more freely than could before the project.

- Student truancy fell.

- Relations between boys and girls in school improved, and the gender gap in aspirations narrowed.

- The number of unplanned pregnancies and abortions declined.

- Students were better able to make informed decisions about reproductive health, STIs, and HIV prevention and complications.

- Empowerment of girls reduced their sexual vulnerability.

The Expanded Life Planning Education Program (ELPE), Nigeria

> The program mainstreamed HIV/AIDS education into the delivery of LPE in schools. This adequately covered provision of information on HIV/AIDS; care and support for People Living Positively and community mobilization activities that discourage stigma and discrimination.
>
> *ELPE Manager*

As the importance of the education sector in HIV prevention has been increasingly recognized, many countries have sought to introduce teaching about HIV as part of a regular school subject. Effecting such a change is challenging. Teachers must be provided with new knowledge and trained in new, participatory ways of teaching. Communities must approve and support changes if they are to be sustainable and effective. Education sectors must be enabled to regulate and manage the teaching of a new subject. Students must adapt to new ways of teaching and learning. How has Nigeria met these challenges?

Description

Nigeria's Expanded Life Planning Education (ELPE) demonstrates how HIV and adolescent reproductive health education can be mainstreamed into the life of schools, teachers, communities, and the education sector to become a normal and everyday part of educational life. The program shows how intersectoral collaboration, community advocacy, effective training of teachers and peer educators, and high-quality research (including monitoring and evaluation) can make the introduction of change acceptable and desirable.

Obatunde Oladapo, consultant, conducted the interviews and collected the data for this chapter. Eccoua Oyinloye, of the Ministry of Education, Science, and Technology, Nigeria, provided support, encouragement, and assistance. Criana Connal, consultant, assisted in drafting the text of this chapter.

Rationale and History

The program was initiated in 1994, when parents and teachers in Ibadan, the capital of Oyo State, raised concerns about the rising incidence of unwanted pregnancy and the death of two girls from septic complications of abortion (figure 9.1). The Association for Reproductive and Family Health (ARFH) was invited to provide life-planning education (LPE) on reproductive health to secondary school students and out-of-school youth.

In 1996 a project was piloted in four secondary schools in Ibadan, with support from the United Kingdom's Overseas Development Agency (ODA). In 1999 the success of the pilot project led to the expansion of activities to 131 secondary schools in the 33 local government areas of the state spanning its eight educational zones. Expansion was supported by the United Kingdom's Department for International Development (DFID), which provided funding for the program from 1999 until 2003.

During the expansion process, various actors were involved in designing the program and its teaching-learning materials. They included government officials, NGO staff, teachers, parents, other community members, and learner representatives. The active involvement of these actors contributed to the fact that the ELPE program has had few real problems in gaining broad acceptance and support.

The rationale underlying the program's activities is as follows:

- Prevention of health problems is far more effective and desirable than treatment.

- The earlier the knowledge and skills to make healthy informed decisions are imparted, the greater are young people's chances of living a healthy lifestyle.

- The school environment is the most appropriate place to provide children, adolescents, and young adults with the opportunity to develop

Figure 9.1: Timeline of ELPE Implementation

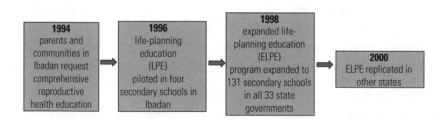

Source: Authors.

knowledge and to adopt healthy attitudes and skills for dealing with life situations.

- Students can learn about how their bodies, especially the reproductive system, work.

- Teachers can be trusted with the task of guiding the behavior of students.

- LPE has the potential to challenge students to take responsibility for their reproductive health behaviors.

- Students feel that classroom teaching of LPE is best. Undertaking LPE in school does most to increase the involvement and participation of students. It captures their attention more and is a more effective means of imparting knowledge and shaping behavior than other (ad hoc) arrangements.

- LPE complements and reinforces other school-based ad hoc initiatives to promote morals and acceptable social behavior.

- Parents believe that classroom delivery of LPE is an effective complement to their own efforts.

Over the years the content of activities has evolved in response to a number of factors:

- Research findings showed that young people in the program area were engaging in risky sexual behaviors that increase the risk of STIs, including HIV infection.

- The incidence of HIV among young people was increasing, intensifying the need to do more to prevent transmission.

- The importance of the home environment—where young people spend more time than at school—and the need to provide parents with more information to enable them to discuss reproductive health issues with their children was recognized.

In response to these factors, ELPE was developed to cover much more than reproductive health education. Topics added to the program included education about the impact of risky sexual behaviors, improved parent/child education, and HIV prevention education.

Since the program's inception, it has gone from a voluntary to a mandatory program in Oyo State. It is officially scheduled in the school timetable and integrated in the Oyo State secondary schools' joint scheme of work (the breakdown of the curriculum into units). The success of the program in Oyo State has led to its replication in Bauchi, Borno Gombe, Kebbi, and Yobe States, with support from the Ford Foundation.

Aim, Objectives, and Strategies

On the contents of the lessons

We are taught about the basic facts about HIV/AIDS; the effects; the causes and how to protect ourselves from being infected. We were taught that HIV is a virus that has no cure. We are also taught how to prevent it especially through abstinence from premarital sex. We are also told how we can avoid HIV and that it is transmitted from mother to her child, through sex and sharing skin-piercing objects with an infected person. They tell us that it is a disease that affects the nation. We are further taught about sexually transmitted infections, teenage pregnancy, its effects and how to avoid it. We are taught how to talk with others, that is communication, and goal setting.

Students at an ELPE school

The main aim of the program is to improve the sexual and reproductive health of in-school youth in Oyo State and to serve as a model for national replication. The program's objectives are as follows:

- Encourage students to develop a positive attitude toward all their bodily functions.

- Increase awareness of the potential consequences of unprotected sex.

- Help students make healthy and informed choices.

- Encourage students to develop relationships based on mutual respect and responsibility.

- Increase students' awareness of cultural and religious influences on relationships and sexuality.

- Encourage better communication about relationships and sexual matters between young people and their parents, guardians, families, and friends.

- Promote the physical, mental, cultural, and spiritual development of students and society, and prepare students for a more responsible adulthood and a smooth transition from adolescence to early adulthood.

- Reinforce the role of parents as a major influence on the growth and development of their children.

The program seeks to meet its objectives through the following strategies:

- Carrying out baseline needs assessment and conducting regular monitoring and evaluation

- Mobilizing and involving parents and communities in various stages of program design and implementation

- Engaging in program advocacy

- Integrating and teaching LPE as a stand-alone subject in the Oyo State secondary school curriculum

- Providing peer education

- Improving access to youth-friendly services.

Target Groups

ELPE's primary target group is students aged 9–20 of both genders and all tribes. The secondary target group includes users of youth-friendly clinics, teachers, parents, and policy makers. The program indirectly targets out-of-school youth (through their in-school peers).

Components

ELPE activities include the following:

- Formal HIV/AIDS education

- Peer education

- LPE and HIV prevention clubs

- Youth-friendly health clinics, set up by the Ministry of Health

- Teacher training

- Material development and distribution

- Research, monitoring, and evaluation

- Advocacy and awareness raising.

Each of these components is discussed in the next section.

Implementation

Partnerships

Program implementation is managed by the program's four key partners, each of which has specific responsibilities. The program's pilot was developed by ARFH in Ibadan, with support from Oyo State's MoEST and Ministry of Health and ODA. In 1999 ELPE became a statutory program in Oyo State, under the responsibility of ARFH; MoEST, Oyo State; the Ministry of Health, Oyo State; and Teaching Service Commission (TESCOM), Oyo State.

ARFH has overall responsibility for the program. Its executive director serves as project coordinator and chief accounting officer.

MoEST has responsibilities for reviewing policy; legalizing and regularizing the integration of LPE into the school curriculum; and strengthening the ministry's approach to the new challenge. The project coordinating unit has responsibilities for other operational issues, such as maintaining links with schools, supervising and monitoring, liaising with other partners, distributing materials to schools, collecting data from schools, providing technical assistance to teachers, setting standards, and ensuring compliance. The project coordinating unit is made up of a team drawn from units of MoEST, including planning, research, and statistics; curriculum development; quality control; and schools.

The Ministry of Health has responsibility for policy review and for facilitating the integration of youth-friendly services into primary health care (Oyo State is one of the few states in Nigeria to provide youth-friendly services within the public health care system). Local government areas and Ministry of Health staff establish youth-friendly units within primary health care centers to provide services to young people. With the support of local government areas, coordinators of primary health care centers monitor and supervise activities at these clinics, reporting their findings to the Ministry of Health. Provision of youth-friendly services is coordinated by a project coordinating unit (made up of people from the planning, research, and statistics units of primary health care centers), which has responsibilities for operational issues, such as maintaining links with local government areas, supervising and monitoring services, liaising with other partners, providing technical assistance to service providers, and collecting data from youth-friendly clinics. As the program moves from being an innovative project to part of the day-to-day work of MoEST, the Ministry of Health is also called upon to provide ongoing support and advice to the educational activities of schools at the local level.

TESCOM is responsible for hiring and transferring teachers. It works to minimize the transfers of teachers selected for LPE training for at least three years during project implementation.

Management Structure

The program operates at the state and local government levels. At the state level, the Project Advisory Committee reviews project implementation, advises on project management, receives feedback, advocates for support for the project, and undertakes oversight functions. It members are drawn from various constituencies—including NGOs, religious groups, professional associations, the public sector (the Nigerian Educational Research and Development Council), and the private sector—bringing rich ideas and different perspectives. The Project Planning and Implementation Team meets monthly to discuss issues, review project implementation, review and draw action plans, and make decisions.

At the local government level, civil servants work with ARFH staff to encourage and enable implementation of LPE in schools and liaise between individual schools and the state MoEST. They are also responsible for supporting supervisors who monitor and evaluate the program. Senior school management implements the program in schools, under the leadership of the school director.

Program Activities

Program activities include formal school activities and peer education. They also include clubs, youth-friendly clinics, and efforts to improve communication between young people and their parents.

Formal school activities

Although LPE is designed to be integrated as a stand-alone unit into the regular curriculum, it is not necessarily delivered in a standard manner in all 131 schools. Depending on the school, LPE is

- taught within the regular curriculum and school timetable, once or twice a week for one hour;

- taught during biology;

- taught as part of literary and debating activities;

- addressed as an extracurricular activity;

- addressed during assembly talks;

- integrated into special events; or

- discussed for at least five minutes a week by various subject teachers.

On being able to set personal goals as a result of ELPE

When I was in Junior Secondary Schools 1 and 2, I did not know how to set my goals, all I had in mind was to achieve something not well-defined in life. Life-planning education has taught me how to set goals and now I have a reading time-table as well. Last term I came first in my class and I made all my papers. I always tell my peers to set their goals properly because it will help them achieve a lot and put them in the right place for the future. As for my friends and me, setting our goals has improved our lives.

Peer Educator, Ibadan

Peer education

ELPE has found the peer education approach to be effective in improving young people's health-seeking behavior and access to reproductive health information. Trained peer educators interact with their peers through discussion, counseling, distribution of materials, dramas, and other means. Peer education takes place during school hours as well as after school. Peer educators counsel and inform their peers on issues relating to adolescent reproductive health and HIV/AIDS. They act under the supervision of LPE teachers (who refer students to youth-friendly clinics when needed). Peer educators take part in the program for as long as they wish to.

> Peer educators communicate in a language that is more likely to be understood [by other young people], they can be a more credible source of information than adult educators. They can serve as positive role models, and identification with them enables students to discuss sensitive issues. At the heart of peer education lie the notions of credibility, trust, and empathy.
>
> *Peer Educator*

> I am proud to be a Peer Educator especially in my school and my street. In addition to applying what I learnt to myself, I have also been able to talk to my peers, friends and other known people in my school and street. And as a result of my activities, I have personally noticed positive changes in my own life and the lives of my friends that usually do some wrong things like following girls up and down, gambling or being rude to teachers or their parents. Also we all now use the time available to us wisely. LPE has also given me room to become a leader because I provide useful information to my age-mates and they respect me. I am able to face people and counsel them—even elderly people like my brother come to me for counseling. LPE has also exposed the secret of the killer disease called HIV/AIDS. I know how it is spread and how to protect myself from it.
>
> *Peer Educator, Ibadan*

Clubs

LPE and HIV prevention clubs meet in schools. They reinforce the teachings of LPE about adolescent reproductive health and issues relating to HIV through discussion, drama, counseling, debating, and other means. Members of the clubs include peer educators and other students. LPE teachers supervise club activities.

Youth-friendly clinics

A component of ELPE is the establishment, by the Ministry of Health, of youth-friendly clinics at local primary health care centers, where young people are able to access reproductive health services, including counseling and treatment for minor ailments, STIs, and other health problems. Trained health providers from these clinics give talks in schools and provide contraceptives, such as condoms, which are not provided in schools.

Student–parent communication

ELPE also aims to improve communication between parents and children. It uses drama, film, and video to facilitate parent–child communication.

Training

Training is provided by staff from ARFH, MoEST, the Ministry of Health, UNICEF, the Society for Family Health, and by consultants from DFID. It consists of training of trainers (two weeks); training of supervisors (two weeks); and training of health care providers (two weeks).

LPE teachers received two weeks and LPE peer educators one week of training, provided at their school by program trainers. LPE teachers were selected based on the recommendation of students, school directors, and ARFH staff, as well as on their educational background, disposition toward students, schedule of duty, and dedication.

The training curriculum for health care providers was divided into six modules: introduction to LPE concepts, adolescent reproductive health issues, adolescent health, communication skills, provision of youth-friendly health services, and management of reproductive health issues.

> **On selecting LPE teachers in schools**
>
> Students were asked to nominate teachers who are firm but friendly and with whom they could relate freely. Educational background, disposition towards young people, sense of duty and dedication were also important. Some teachers were recommended by principals and members of staff.
>
> *Program Implementers*

Training of teachers

The objectives of teacher training are to:

- empower teachers to provide sex education that equips students to make informed decisions and improve their social and sexual behaviors

- enable teachers to implement HIV interventions in various communities (schools, rural areas, and so forth)

- facilitate the effective and judicious delivery of LPE in schools.

Training covers a range of topics, including the following:

- What LPE is

- Needs assessment and baseline survey

- Value clarification

- Adolescent reproductive health

- Gender issues

- Anatomy and physiology

- Teenage pregnancy

- Substance abuse

- STIs, including HIV

- Poverty reduction

- Relationships

- Life-building skills

- Communication, negotiation, self-esteem, study skills, goal setting, and related topics

- Counseling

- Participatory learning and action

- Monitoring and evaluation

- Community mobilization.

LPE teachers are trained using participatory teaching-learning methods, providing them the opportunity to experience these methods themselves. These methods included the following:

- Discussions

- Brainstorming

- Group work

- Experiential learning and models

- Demonstrations, role-plays, lectures, facilitated discussions, dramas, questioning, real-life stories, and singing.

A two-day refresher training for staff is conducted periodically to:

- refresh and update knowledge of topics taught during training

- consider the challenges faced and try to find solutions to them

- allow teachers' experience to inform the work of program designers and evaluators.

Training of peer educators

Staff of ARFH, teachers, and students selected the peer educators, on the basis of their popularity, ability to communicate with peers, leadership qualities, integrity, conduct, and regular attendance at school. Peer educators were chosen from junior-secondary 1 and 2 and senior-secondary 1 and 2 (that is, they were not in their last year of either junior- or senior-secondary school). More than 2,500 young people were trained as peer educators in this manner. An important aspect of selection was gender equality.

The objectives of training were to enable peer educators to:

- increase their knowledge of adolescent sexuality, reproductive health, and HIV/AIDS issues and acquire the skills needed to help them solve problems and pass knowledge on to peers

- advise peers on reproductive health issues

- act as counselors and role models

- disseminate information to out-of-school peers

- introduce students in other schools to LPE

- influence their peers positively.

Topics covered during training of peer educators included the following:

- Who is a peer educator?

- Adolescent reproductive and sexual health

- Sexuality, society, and culture

- Values and values clarification

- STIs, HIV/AIDS, gender issues, life-planning skills, beating poverty, menstruation, conception, teenage pregnancy and abortion, human anatomy and physiology, counseling, substance abuse, and related issues

As in teacher training, participatory teaching-learning methods were used, allowing peer educators to experience and become familiar with the methods before using some of them in their interaction with peers.

Curricular Approach, Time Allocation, and Assessment

The focus of teaching-learning was initially on core life-planning topics. As it became apparent how serious the problem of HIV/AIDS was, the focus shifted to age-appropriate HIV prevention education, provided through:

- drama, songs, dance, role-plays, storytelling, group discussions, and presentations

- projects, cultural displays, workshops, assembly talks, and seminars

- local excursions to places of interest, such as youth-friendly clinics, and community outreach activities

- peer counseling and referrals to youth-friendly health centers.

Different kinds of activities are used to achieve different learning objectives. Peer counseling is used to positively influence students' attitudes. Presentations and role-play are used to build skills. Group discussion and information, education, and communication materials are used to build knowledge.

The topics covered during LPE lessons include the following:

- Communication skills

- Peer pressure and how to deal with it

- Sexuality, society, and culture

- Human growth and development

- STIs and HIV/AIDS

- Prevention of pregnancy

- Self-esteem

- Child rights, including the right to say no to sex

- Negotiation and decision-making skills

- Sexual violence

- Self-assessment of risk of HIV infection

- Poverty-reduction/income-generation skill building

- Time management.

Teaching covers how HIV infection does and does not occur, HIV prevalence rates in Nigeria, signs and symptoms of HIV/AIDS, caring for people living with HIV/AIDS, misconceptions about HIV/AIDS, and how to protect oneself from HIV, including through abstinence and safe sex. Students are provided with information on condom use and referred to youth-friendly health centers, where condoms are supposed to be available.

Implementers' comments on pedagogical approach

ELPE emphasizes training as opposed to teaching. Also the participatory learning and action approaches employed in the delivery of ELPE make application of knowledge possible. Learning is by doing, so by implication, in ELPE generally—including the delivery of sessions on HIV/AIDS, the 3 domains of knowledge are emphasized, that is, knowledge, attitude and psycho-motoric. So, a strong connection of theory and practice exists in the teaching of HIV/AIDS.

In Oyo State, much of what is taught is theory because the syllabus is followed. I make it a participatory learning and action system by showing activities of the issue, for example, inviting PLWHA, PABA and vulnerable children to participate in programs whenever the opportunity arises.

ELPE Implementers

Materials

ARFH produced the ELPE program materials in collaboration with project partners and other stakeholders, including MoEST, the Ministry of Health, the National Education Research and Development Council, teachers, students, counselors, youths, and NGOs, with financial support from DFID. Materials were produced in Yoruba and English. Design of the materials was influenced by a variety of factors, including the findings of the needs assessment, the cultural background of the target audience, available resources, prevailing issues, students' ideas and views, and requests. Using the findings of the needs assessment and baseline survey, program officials developed materials that provide LPE teachers and peer educators with the support needed to implement the LPE lessons and activities; information on adolescent reproductive health issues; and answers to a range of questions that "had been bothering students."

A range of real-life stories and case studies was included in the curriculum; the information, education, and communication materials; and the manuals. Teaching aids, such as charts, were designed to ease learning and to make it more interesting. (As the implementers say, "Children love picture reading.")

Manual for trainers

The trainers' manual covers areas such as values and value clarification, the anatomy of male and female reproductive organs, life-planning skills, poverty-reducing strategies, relationships, puberty, and adolescence.

Materials for use by teachers

The LPE syllabus was produced by ARFH in collaboration with MoEST, the Ministry of Health, LPE teachers, students, and researchers. This 223-page document guides teachers in delivering LPE lessons. It sets out the scope of what is to be taught at each level and provides information about session objectives, teaching methods, and the use of instructional materials.

A teachers' handbook provides teachers with additional information about adolescent reproductive issues. Topics covered included basic anatomy and physiology, life-planning skills, STIs, HIV/AIDS, adolescence, teenage pregnancy, and related issues.

On the use of case studies in the teaching materials

Many true life stories and case studies that relate to the students were included in the curriculum, the information, education, and communication materials and manuals. As a result, students easily relate the issues to their own ways of life.

LPE Implementer

A helpful addition for teachers was the provision of hard-board, spiral-bound flipcharts with tricolor illustrations for use during training, counseling, and teaching of LPE. The flipcharts cover male and female anatomy and physiology, HIV/AIDS education, gender issues, and related issues.

Handbook for peer educators

The handbook provides peer educators with information on male and female reproductive systems, negotiating, coping with peer pressure, values and value clarification, effective communication, study skills, sexuality, STIs, the rights of the child, HIV/AIDS, and voluntary counseling and testing.

Materials for use by young people

This manual is a 153-page document designed to help in-school and out-of-school youth learn about sexuality and life-planning skills. It covers topics such as knowing oneself, making good choices, sexual health, and sexuality as the fabric of life. The manual was produced by ARFH, in association with Advocates for Youth, a Washington, DC–based NGO. The manual is accompanied by a workbook that enables students to follow topics taught during LPE sessions.

A biannual magazine (*Youthscope*) was also produced for students. It contained articles about life skills, sexuality, reproduction, and family health.

Monitoring and referral forms

Monitoring forms are designed for use by teachers and peer educators. The forms are to be used on a weekly, monthly, and quarterly basis to assess implementation of LPE activities. They monitor the number of boys and girls taking part in activities, challenges educators are confronted with, lessons learned, and other issues. The referral forms are designed for use by peer educators to facilitate quick referral to health care services when necessary.

Information, education, and communication materials

The program has produced a wide range of information, education, and communication materials for use in schools, including posters, leaflets, tracts, films, videos, pictures, and magazines. Titles include "Stay Away from Drugs"; "Help, Help, Help, before HIV/AIDS Destroys Our Nation"; "Stop Sexual Abuse, Speak Out"; and "Good Study Habits."

Assessment of Students

There is no formal or systematic evaluation of learning. Teachers and peer educators monitor progress through periodic completion of the monitoring forms. Teachers also assess students' progress by asking questions informally, by assessing student assignments, and by evaluating inputs from peer educators and community members.

Advocacy

Advocacy is an important part of the ELPE program. It seeks to ensure support for and acceptability of the program by a range of key political actors as well as school personnel. Advocacy has helped sustain and expand the program.

Advocacy to influence policy makers

Sensitization of policy makers and community leaders has occurred in a number of ways. Early on, key program officials paid courtesy visits to the

ministries of education and health, to familiarize staff there with the objectives of the program. Advocacy meetings—including briefings and consultative meetings for policy makers in the education and health ministries—
are held regularly at the local, state, and federal levels.

In March 1998, before the program was scaled up, a stakeholders' and
strategy review conference was held. The meeting enabled key stakeholders
to provide input on project implementation and expansion. It was attended
by more than 250 key stakeholders, including representatives of the state
ministries of health and education; donor organizations; NGOs; teachers
and principals; representatives of the All Nigerian Conference of Principals
of Secondary Schools and the Nigerian Union of Teachers; parents;
students and out-of-school youth; and religious leaders.

In 2003, following the program's evaluation (described below), the findings, lessons learned, and challenges faced were discussed with federal
government officials. The meeting was attended by policy makers from
about 22 states.

Advocacy in schools

Orientation sessions were held in every project school, with the aim of
informing school staff about the program aims and strategies and building
support within the school, in particular the support of principals. During
implementation of the program, it was found that LPE teachers and peer
educators were being bullied by non–LPE teachers and students (in the case
of peer educators, whose commitment to the program actually increased as
a result). Additional program advocacy activities conducted in schools were
conducted to help non–LPE teachers understand and accept ELPE activities and to support teachers and peer educators in their efforts to implement
ELPE activities.

Advocacy for greater involvement by communities

From its inception, ELPE has actively sought to involve all stakeholders.
The advice and support of community leaders have been sought at all stages
of the program. Community leaders are invited to all ELPE activities
organized by schools. To ease acceptance of program content, the program
used culturally acceptable terminology. It has also tried to mobilize community members to discourage stigma and discrimination.

Acceptance of the program by parents and guardians was crucial, for two
reasons. First, parents and guardians can complement the school-based

LPE education by talking with their children about related issues at home. Second, parents who oppose the program can prevent their children from taking part in LPE activities (parents' permission for students' participation in LPE activities is always sought). Parental involvement took place during different stages of program development and implementation, including the needs assessment/baseline survey, stakeholders' conference, and interim evaluation.

Community advocacy strategies have included the following:

- Convening of advocacy meetings with community opinion leaders and religious leaders

- Use of interviews and focus group discussions during program design processes

- Broadcasting of radio and television jingles

- Broadcasting of dramas and mini-dramas on television

- Inclusion of LPE talks at PTA meetings

- Organization of road shows, outreach efforts, mini-conferences, informal seminars, films, concerts, and drama presentations.

Results of advocacy

When the program began, it encountered resistance from religious leaders and others. Since then advocacy activities have led to wide acceptance of the program. Advocacy measures have resulted in the following:

- Establishment of LPE coordinating units in the ministries of education and health

- Integration of LPE into the curriculum and timetable, so that it is now taught as a required subject in secondary schools in Oyo State

- Acceptance of and cooperation with the program by communities

- Replication of the program in other states in Nigeria.

Costs

During the period 1999–2003, ELPE benefited about 425,000 young people and 7,000 adults, at a cost of less than $800,000 ($1.78 per person) (tables 9.1 and 9.2).

Table 9.1: Annual Costs of ELPE, 1999–2003

(U.S. dollars)

YEAR	AMOUNT
1999	162,000
2000	169,000
2001	277,000
2002	133,000
2003	26,000
Total	767,000

Source: ARFH.

Table 9.2: Cost of ELPE, 1999–2003, by Category

(U.S. dollars)

CATEGORY	AMOUNT
Training	340,000
Salaries	146,000
Research and evaluation	93,000
Information, education, and communication; advocacy; and community development	58,000
Refurbishment and equipment of youth-friendly clinics[a]	45,000
Institutional development	31,000
Curriculum review	17,000
Administration	16,000
Monitoring and supervision	12,000
Other	9,000
Total	767,000

Source: ARFH.

a. The program had two components—the greater was teaching in schools (led by MoE), the lesser was the establishment of youth-friendly services at health centers (led by MoH).

Monitoring and Evaluation

M&E is an integral part of ELPE. To scale up the program effectively, ARFH conducted a needs assessment in Oyo State in 1998. The assessment occurred in all 33 local government areas, spanning the state's eight educational zones. The assessment was undertaken by a multi-disciplinary team, coordinated by ARFH's Evaluation and Operations Research Department.

Both quantitative and qualitative data were collected from all 131 project schools. Participatory learning and action methods (including focus group discussions and questionnaires completed by teachers, parents, and students) were used to collect qualitative data. Use of participatory learning and action enabled all stakeholders to share their opinions on the project concept. Data were collected from 25 students and 14 teachers per school, principals and vice-principals of each school, 20 parents per school locality, and selected other individuals from communities (table 9.3).

The needs assessment revealed several important findings:

- A sizable percentage of young people are sexually active and do not possess the necessary knowledge to safeguard themselves against potential problems associated with sex. Early pregnancy and abortion are common.

- The main sources of reproductive health information are peers, the media, and health workers (in this order).

- Young people rely most on their peers to help them resolve problems.

- Young people's preferred sources of reproductive health information are health providers; (older, married) teachers; older siblings; parents; and friends.

- Young people's sources of reproductive health treatment are patent medicine dealers, traditional healers, self-medication, and government health centers.

- Poverty is a major cause of risky reproductive health behavior.

- Parents and teachers see themselves as incapable of offering solutions to adolescent reproductive health problems.

- Sexual abuse of children by adults, including teachers, is common.

This information represented a baseline against which project performance was periodically assessed. Measurable indicators were developed in a collaborative effort by the Ministry of Health, MoEST, ARFH, and DFID. The findings were used to design implementation strategies, including the LPE curriculum.

An implementer's view on the results of the needs' assessment:

- Adolescent boys and girls are sexually active
- Early pregnancy was rampant
- Abortion was common among girls
- Teacher-student relationship was being abused
- All stakeholders desired action
- All stakeholders were tired (of the situation) and helpless
- Moral laxity in schools and the society
- Adolescents get wrong information about sexuality
- Parents have shirked their responsibilities (to their children)

ELPE Implementer

Table 9.3: Assessment Information Collected from Student, Teacher, and Parent Questionnaires

STUDENTS	TEACHERS	PARENTS
Demographic information	Demographic information	Demographic information
Living arrangements	Observed changes in students	Person responsible for paying school
Person responsible for	Knowledge of students' reproductive	fees
meeting students' needs	health problems	Perceptions of problems confronting
Spare-time interests	Perception of students' coping mechanisms	students
Concerns and problems	Reasons for drop-out	Specific reproductive health problems
Gender-related issues	Disciplinary action taken against	of male and female youth
Planned age of marriage	pregnant girl and partner	Community's attempt to solve
Planned number of children	Knowledge of students who have	adolescent reproductive health
Knowledge and discussion of	had abortions	problems
reproductive health issues with	Opinion about use of contraceptives	Avenues through which young people's
others	by young people	social and financial needs are met
Sources of information on reproductive	Awareness of youth-friendly clinic	Rate of drop-out and withdrawal
health issues	in locality	from school and reasons
Sexual experience and behavior	Perception of teacher-student relationship	Awareness of contraceptives and
Reproductive health topics	(including sexual)	attitude toward their use by
students would want information on	Perception of stakeholders' participation	young people

Source: ARFH.

Monitoring

Program monitoring and supervision takes place at four levels:

- Level 1: Each school selects an LPE coordinator, who supervises daily activities. He or she oversees and supervises the activities of other LPE teachers. The principal is responsible for ensuring that LPE teaching is conducted regularly, according to the agreed schedule.

- Level 2: Zonal and local education inspectors monitor the activities of LPE teachers monthly.

- Level 3: MoEST (the project coordinating unit) monitors the first and second levels on a bimonthly basis.

- Level 4: Program partners (ARFH, MoEST, and the Ministry of Health) jointly supervise program implementation on a quarterly basis.

Both teachers and peer educators were equipped with monitoring and referral forms. These forms were filled out weekly, monthly, and quarterly as a means of monitoring peer educators' and teachers activities. Responses enabled information to be gathered about the gender distribution of activities, challenges, lessons learned, and expected outcomes.

LPE teachers in each school regularly meet to discuss progress and challenges. They hold joint meetings with peer educators every two weeks, mainly to discuss and find solutions to problems peer educators encounter.

In 2001 the LPE teachers' forum was set up. LPE teachers meet to exchange ideas and experiences with regard to implementing LPE lessons in schools.

Evaluation

Conducting evaluations and making use of their findings was one of the main strategies of the program. Evaluations were undertaken to detect changes in knowledge, attitudes, and behaviors by stakeholders; investigate the process, lessons, challenges, and outcomes of the program; and assist others in replicating the program.

The survey was readministered during a "process" evaluation in 2001–03 and an "outcome" evaluation in 2003, when DFID funding ended. Students, teachers, principals, health providers, religious leaders, and parents were asked to respond to questions about:

- major reproductive health and nonreproductive health issues facing students

- student knowledge of reproductive health issues and issues associated with maturing

- students' social and sexual behavior

- students' perspectives on and concerns about issues that have direct and indirect bearings on them

- students' ability to deal with peer pressure, their use of leisure time, and their preferred sources of information on reproductive health and HIV/AIDS

- parents' perspectives on reproductive health and other issues relating directly and indirectly to their children

- the place of LPE in the life of schools

- teachers' perspectives on students' social and sexual behavior

- types of services and support system available for meeting identified needs

- preferences of different stakeholders for different strategies for resolving problems

- health providers' knowledge, attitude, and practice of adolescent reproductive health issues and services and their opinion about access to such services

- the quality of health facilities in the community.

The assessment revealed several important findings:

- Young people can be change agents if their talents, skills, and energies are properly channeled.

- Peer education is effective in empowering young people in public speaking, interpersonal communication, counseling, decision making, problem solving, and development of leadership skills. It also improves health-seeking behavior and access to reproductive health information.

- ELPE allowed students to discuss reproductive health issues with their teachers more freely.

- The level of truancy dropped (according to both focus group discussions and surveys).

- The relationship between boys and girls in school improved, with the gap in aspirations closing as LPE expanded the horizons of both male and female students.

- The number of unplanned pregnancies and abortions fell.

- Patronage of youth-friendly clinics increased. The majority of health providers remarked that students were more open about their reproductive health problems than before the program and were able to make informed choices.

- Empowerment of girls reduced their sexual vulnerability.

Based on these findings, adjustments were made to the program, placing more emphasis on teaching and learning about HIV/AIDS, for example.

Lessons Learned

Implementation of the program revealed several challenges. It also yielded lessons about how to deal with them.

Government/NGO Cultures

In the process of implementation, it became apparent that substantive differences existed between the NGO and the ministries with respect to matters such as structures and administration. The bureaucratic nature of the civil service was found to be at odds with the pragmatic approach of the NGO. These differences sometimes led to tension and conflict.

The program worked hard to bring the ministries and the NGO together. Regular and effective communication and a willingness on all sides to be patient were essential. Effective advocacy led to political commitment to program aims. The NGO also introduced training to transfer program management skills to the ministries.

Teacher Transfer

An initial challenge encountered by the program was the interruption of LPE teaching as a result of the frequent transfer of LPE-trained teachers to schools that did not offer the course. The fact that donor agencies and NGOs often hire LPE–trained teachers as consultants also poses a challenge to the continuity of the program (while attesting to its merit).

The challenge of the frequent transfer of teachers was resolved by bringing members of TESCOM into the Project Implementation Team. TESCOM worked to minimize the transfer of trained LPE teachers.

Managers tend to view the second challenge—the hiring of LPE teachers as consultants—as a considerable accolade for the program. It should nevertheless be flagged as a potential concern for the program's viability.

Taking LPE Seriously

When LPE was first introduced, students sometimes approached the subject with less seriousness than they did subjects on which they are examined. The program responded to students' attitude in a number of ways. LPE is now on the school timetable and the Oyo State secondary schools' joint scheme of work. The participatory approach to teaching has done much to sustain students' interest, and continuous advocacy has sustained support for the program.

Sustainability

DFID provided funds for the scaling up of ELPE between 1999 and 2003, when external funding ended. Now that DFID funding is no longer being provided, program officials must ensure that sufficient funding is available to ensure the program continues and that LPE teachers are replaced when they leave their schools.

Part of the challenge of program sustainability is the overcrowded curriculum and overstretched teachers. LPE is designed to be taught as a stand-alone subject for about one hour a week, but teachers indicate they do not have enough time to effectively teach the subject. Schools and teachers often have to be creative in finding the time to cover LPE topics within the overcrowded school program.

The government of Oyo has expressed enthusiasm for the program to be continued and has supported the integration of LPE into the school curriculum. Project staff have sought to integrate LPE into the curricula of federal and state colleges of education so that all new teachers can deliver the subject. Increasing the number of teachers trained in LPE could improve LPE teaching and learning. However, not all teachers are able to effectively discuss issues relating to sexuality. Much will depend on ensuring that students feel comfortable talking to teachers about such issues.

Poverty and Commercial Sex Work

Poverty leads many girls to have sex for money, putting them at higher risk of HIV and other STIs. Parents are unable to prevent this from happening, because they are not able to meet the needs of their children themselves. In some cases parents and guardians encourage the practice, to bring more income into the family.

Poverty lies at the heart of the spread and impact of HIV. To address the problem, the program included strategies to reduce poverty in the LPE syllabus. By doing so, the program aims to help girls find alternative means of earning income. Strengthening girls' negotiating skills helps them reject sexual advances by adults, including teachers.

Conclusion

ELPE has become an accepted part of secondary education in Oyo State, as a result of a number of factors. First, the development of the program was based on high-quality research. Second, the program engages in intense and effective advocacy. Third, the program created successful partnerships and garnished the support of politicians, schools, teachers, and communities. The program's success—and replication in other states—shows the value of school-based HIV prevention.

Annex 9.1

ELPE Attainment of Impact Benchmarks

BENCHMARK	ATTAINMENT/COMMENTS
1. Identifies and focuses on specific sexual health goals	✓
2. Focuses narrowly on specific behaviors that lead to sexual health goals	✓
3. Identifies and focuses on sexual psychosocial risk and protective factors that are highly related to each of these behaviors	✓ Program promotes the physical, mental, cultural, and spiritual development of students and society; it prepares students for a more responsible adulthood and a smoother transition from adolescence to early adulthood.
4. Implements multiple activities to change each of the selected risk and protective factors	✓ Program uses a wide range of strategies, including teaching in different subject areas, school health clubs, peer educators, outreach to the community.
5. Actively involves youth by creating a safe social environment	✓ Intense advocacy in communities helps teachers enable young people to address various issues, knowing that their teaching is supported by parents and the community. LPE teachers often begin a session using humor, to create a positive climate. Learners' questions are welcomed.
6. Employs a variety of teaching methods designed to involve participants and have them personalize the information	✓
7. Conveys clear message about sexual activity and condom or contraceptive use and continually reinforces that message	✓ The program provides clear information about abstinence, safer sex practices, and negotiation and refusal skills. Trained health providers from youth-friendly clinics give talks in schools and provide students with condoms, which are not provided in schools.
8. Includes effective curricula and activities appropriate to the age, sexual experience, and culture of participating students	✓ Research ensures that curricula and messages are tailored to the circumstances and reality of students.
9. Increases knowledge by providing basic, accurate information about the risks of teen sexual activity and methods of avoiding intercourse or using protection against pregnancy and STIs	✓ Course content on HIV is strong and clear.
10. Uses some of the same strategies to change perceptions of peer values, to recognize peer pressure to have sex, and to address that pressure	✓ Program evaluation showed that use of peer educators was particularly effective in helping students address peer issues.
11. Identifies specific situations that might lead to sex, unwanted sex, or unprotected sex and identifies methods of avoiding those situations or getting out of them	✓ Role-plays, dramas, and anonymous question boxes enabled students to identify situations that might lead to sexual encounters and help them avoid them. Evaluation indicates that girls' empowerment has been particularly effective in allowing them to reject sex.
12. Provides modeling of and practice with communication, negotiation, and refusal skills to improve both skills and self-efficacy in using those skills	✓ Life-skills content of curriculum encourages students to learn and use communication, negotiation, and refusal skills.

Source: Authors.

Annex 9.2

Contact Information

Mrs. G. E. Delano, Executive Director
Expanded Life Planning Education
Association for Reproductive and Family Health
Qtr 815 A, Army Officers' Mess Road
Agodi GRA Ikolaba
P. O. Box 30259
Ibadan, Nigeria

National Family Life HIV/AIDS Education Curriculum Implementation at a Glance

Description: Curriculum-based HIV/AIDS and life-skills program in junior-secondary schools in Lagos State

Number of schools participating: 334

Coverage: About 42 percent of public junior-secondary schools in Lagos State, reaching 320,000 young people. About 1,650 carrier subject teachers and 100 staff members of the Lagos State Ministry of Education (LSMoE) received training.

Target groups: Students aged 9–13 in public junior-secondary school. Secondary target group includes policy makers, principals, and parents.

Components: The program includes six components:

- Creating supportive environments and increasing stakeholders' knowledge and understanding

- Increasing LSMoE's capacity to implement the program

- Providing in-school education

- Developing materials

- Disseminating information and providing technical support for scaling up the program

- Monitoring and evaluating results.

Establishment and duration: Meetings between the NGO Action Health Incorporated (AHI) and LSMoE began in 2000; a planning meeting was held in January 2003. Classroom delivery began in October 2003. By the end of 2004, implementation had commenced in the more than 300 public junior-secondary schools in the state.

Management: Coordinated by LSMoE, which also advocates for and partially funds program implementation (paying all teacher salaries)

Role of partners: AHI provides technical and financial support. The Lagos State AIDS Control Agency; the Ford, MacArthur, and Packard Foundations; and the World Bank provided additional support at key moments.

Costs: $2.58 per student over three years

Chapter 10

Key evaluation results: Evaluation indicates improvements in students':

- knowledge of how to protect their health
- respect for one another's rights to delay the onset of sexual activity
- communication skills
- grasp of the vocabulary of sexuality and health
- understanding of meaning and desirability of abstinence
- knowledge of personal hygiene
- awareness of the risk of early pregnancy.

Teachers were generally positive about the curriculum but were still struggling to apply life-skills-building teaching methods.

The National Family Life HIV/AIDS Education Curriculum Implementation Program, Lagos State, Nigeria

Curriculum-based teaching about HIV/AIDS has the potential to reach school-age children at the national scale. Nigeria's Family Life HIV/AIDS Education (FLHE) Curriculum Implementation Program is an example of one way in which partnerships between government and civil society can reach a large number of young people with comprehensive prevention and life-skills education.

Description

The government of Lagos State prides itself on the success of the FLHE program, which reaches about 320,000 young people a year. A testament to the efficacy of the program is the fact that the National Council on Education (the country's highest decision-making body on education) approved the program's curriculum for integration into the regular curriculum across Nigeria, as reflected in the 2003 revision of the national policy on education.

Rationale and History

Development of the FLHE program took place over a period of four years. Between 2000 and 2003, advocacy and consultative meetings were held with various stakeholders, including the Lagos State AIDS Control Agency, the Parent-Teacher Association, the National Union of Teachers,

Toyin Akpan, consultant, conducted the interviews and collected the data for this chapter. Nike Esiet, Executive Director/CEO, AHI; Uwem Esiet, Director, AHI; and Bunmi Olatunde (consultant) provided support, encouragement, and assistance.

the All-Nigerian Conference of Principals of Secondary Schools, the State Primary-School Board, the Conference of Primary-School Headmasters of Nigeria, government officials in the education sector, professionals in the higher education sector, religious leaders, and people in the media.

The program was developed on the basis of the results of a needs assessment conducted in 23 public junior-secondary schools in Lagos State in November 2002, as well as findings from other studies and surveys (such as the Demographic and Health Survey). The results of the studies clearly demonstrated a strong need for education on sexual and reproductive health, HIV/AIDS, and other STIs. A planning meeting for program implementation was held in January 2003. Materials were then developed and implementation begun in October 2003 in 100 pilot public junior-secondary schools in Lagos State. Between 2003 and 2004 FLHE was introduced in more than 300 public junior-secondary schools in the state.

Aims, Objectives, and Strategies

The main aim of the program is to meet the sexual and reproductive health needs of 9- to 13-year-old students in Lagos State. Its objectives are to:

- increase the age of first intercourse and marriage

- reduce the rate of teenage pregnancy

- reduce the rate of STI and HIV infection

- reduce the stigmatization associated with HIV/AIDS.

The program seeks to meet its objectives by:

- providing information about sexuality and HIV/AIDS

- helping students clarify attitudes and values that promote good health and behavior

- helping students develop the interpersonal skills they need to safeguard their health

- training students to exercise responsibility when making decisions.

Target Groups

The primary target of FLHE is students in the first three years of public junior-secondary school (9- to 13-year-olds). Secondary target groups include target policy makers, principals, and parents, whose support is crucial to the success of the program.

Approaches

The program is based on the principle that the best way to curb the spread of HIV among children and youth in Nigeria is through a comprehensive school-based program. It is also based on an understanding that the better educated children are, the better able they are to use their knowledge, skills, and confidence to protect themselves against HIV.

The program seeks to provide young people with a comprehensive program that is accessible, nonjudgmental, and responsive to their needs. The provision of FLHE education within the regular school curriculum is considered an important part of this comprehensive response. It allows large numbers of in-school adolescents to be reached at a low cost to the government.

The program is implemented through participatory classroom sessions. It addresses factors that affect HIV transmission, including personal behavior and skills, relationships, community norms and values, and gender issues. It also provides accurate and useful information on sexuality and reproductive health and encourages students to take responsibility for their actions. Teaching-learning sessions include activities such as role-play and other skill-building activities and group discussions issues such as peer pressure, changes during puberty, teenage pregnancy, gender, and abstinence.

Components

The program consists of six components, which build on and complement one another:

- Creating supportive environments and increasing stakeholders' knowledge and understanding
- Increasing LSMoE's capacity to implement the program
- Providing in-school education
- Developing materials
- Disseminating information and providing technical support for scaling up the program
- Monitoring and evaluating results.

Implementation

In the course of program implementation, two changes were made. The first was the title, which was changed from "Sexuality Education" to

"Family Life and HIV Education." The second was the content of the program. Many parents, politicians, and religious leaders found the program's original curriculum—which included discussion of condoms, contraception, and masturbation—too explicit. These and other controversial issues were therefore removed from the curriculum. While the revised curriculum did not contain everything its planners had intended to include, compromise ensured that many of its original objectives continued to be met.

In-School Education

The main component of the program is classroom sessions, which form an integral part of the regular school timetable. FLHE lessons take place three times a week in all public junior-secondary schools in the state.

Skills-building activities are incorporated into lessons and include topics such as negotiation, communication, decision-making, and goal-setting skills; and ways to resist peer influence, reduce risk, and prevent HIV.

Materials

The Ministry of Education and the NGO Action Health Incorporated (AHI) collaborated on the development of curricula on family life and HIV/AIDS education.[1] These curricula were approved by the National Council on Education for use in schools. The development of the national FLHE curriculum was led by three key institutions: the Nigerian Education Research and Development Council (NERDC), the federal Ministry of Education, and AHI. A range of other groups and individuals—including academics, state ministries of education, civil society organizations (CSOs), and religious groups—also contributed to development and review of the curriculum.

A range of English-language materials was developed between 1999 and 2004, including materials for teachers, teacher trainers, and program developers. The development of program materials was based on:

- requests by teachers and program implementers

- the overall goals and objectives of the program

- adaptation of six key concepts from guidelines for comprehensive sexuality education in Nigeria

- cultural norms and values

- age appropriateness

- the educational level of the target audience.

Materials developed included the following:

- Comprehensive Sexuality Education Trainers' Resource Manual

- National Family Life and HIV Education Curriculum for Junior-Secondary School in Nigeria (revised version of the National Comprehensive Sexuality Education Curriculum for Junior, Senior, and Tertiary Institutions in Nigeria)

- Integrated scheme of work for FLHE

- Comprehensive Sexuality Education Trainers' Resource Manual

- Laminated cardboard posters to be used as teaching aids.

Comprehensive sexuality education trainers' resource manual

This manual is used as a reference document by teachers, teacher trainers, and other professionals working in the field. All FLHE-trained teachers and state personnel in Lagos State have been given copies. Teachers in other states in Nigeria also use the material.

The manual provides a step-by-step guide to teaching the topics in the FLHE curriculum as well as other issues. It provides guidelines on how to set the tone in the classroom, deal with sensitive topics, keep parents and caregivers informed, and related issues. It addresses topics such as relationships; human development; sexual health and behavior; skills; and sexuality, society, and culture. Additional information is provided to help teachers answer questions students may pose.

National family life and HIV education curriculum

The curriculum was developed through a participatory process facilitated by NERDC, the federal Ministry of Education, and AHI. To ensure sociocultural appropriateness, curriculum development drew on the perspectives of resource people from the five geopolitical zones of Nigeria.

For each age group, the curriculum identifies the topics to be addressed, the performance objectives, the core contents, the activities to be conducted, and the teaching and learning materials to be used. A copy of the FLHE curriculum is available in each junior-secondary school. Teachers across the country use it as a guide when developing their lessons.

Integrated scheme of work for FLHE

The LSMoE Curriculum Department, in cooperation with teachers, AHI, and other experts, developed the integrated scheme of work for FLHE. It is used as a weekly guideline for teaching FLHE as an integrated topic within the two carrier subjects. The scheme of work presents a sequential list of topics that should be taught each week in all junior grades in the state.

Comprehensive sexuality education trainers' resource manual

This manual was created for the original sexuality education curriculum and covers the full range of topics of that curriculum. It is used by teachers as a resource should students raise issues not covered by the revised FLHE curriculum, such as condom usage.

Posters

LSMoE, AHI, and teachers prepared a range of posters for junior-secondary school teachers in Lagos. Teachers are expected to use these colorful posters to support teaching-learning. Topics addressed by the posters include physical changes during puberty, how HIV/AIDS is and is not spread, non-stereotypical roles (gender roles), menstruation and fertilization, and tips on healthy living.

Training

The training component of the program targets carrier subject teachers and master trainers. Education on FHLE is also being integrated into tertiary teacher education at the preservice level. It is expected that the National Universities Commission, which sets standards for all universities in the federation; the National Commission for Colleges of Education, which sets standards for teacher education; and the National Teachers' Institute, which supervises teachers' in-service activities, will mainstream the FHLE curriculum in the schools they supervise. The Adeniran Ogunsanya College of Education, the Lagos State College of Primary Education, and Lagos State University have integrated FLHE into their preservice training courses.

Teacher training

Training focuses on three areas: technical content; teachers' comfort level in teaching about sexuality; and teaching methodologies appropriate to the core learning domains (cognitive, affective, and behavioral). It seeks to increase teachers':

- knowledge in the areas of sexuality most relevant in the FLHE program

- understanding of their role in providing FLHE

- ability to facilitate learning activities using participatory and experiential learning activities, respond to questions and provide sources for accurate information, respond respectfully and nonjudgmentally to comments reflecting values different from their own, and adapt training to meet the diverse needs of students.

During the pilot phase, 200 teachers of carrier subjects were selected from 100 randomly selected public schools. No more than two teachers from the same school were chosen for training. Selection was based on years of teaching experience (at least three); location (to ensure representation from each senatorial district); and type of school (to ensure balanced representation from model, upgraded, and general schools; rural and urban schools; and single-sex and co-ed schools).

A core group of trainers and one master trainer selected by AHI facilitated the two-week training workshops. The workshops were conducted between May and September 2003, with each workshop training 35 teachers. All groups received the same training.[2] Between February and June 2005, all remaining teachers of integrated science and social studies were trained.

AHI conducted the first set of trainings of 200 teachers. LSMoE conducted the training of another 200 teachers, with technical support from AHI. LSMoE master trainers trained by AHI then facilitated the training of 1,250 teachers. AHI provided general oversight for coordination of master trainers' activities; LSMoE staff from the Inspectorate and the Post Primary Teaching Service Commission (PP TESCOM) (renamed the Teachers Establishment and Pensions Office [TEPO]) coordinated training logistics.

The training workshop lasted 10 working days. The first 5 days consisted of classroom sessions, in which participatory learning approaches were used. The next 4 days were devoted to teaching practice. Each trainee was given a topic to teach; participants took turns teaching the class, with a trained teacher supervising. The last day was devoted to a review.

Topics covered in the training included the following:

- Goals and key concepts in FLHE

- Adolescence

- Facilitation techniques

- What gets in the way of talking comfortably about sexuality

- Values and values clarification

- Gender issues

- Qualities of an effective FLHE teacher

- Communication

- Dealing with hard-to-teach topics

- Teaching aids/sourcing for materials

- Anatomy and physiology

- Defining sex and sexuality over the life cycle

- HIV/AIDS

- Care and support for people living with HIV/AIDS

- Principles of adolescent sexuality counseling

- Teaching practice

The training used a variety of methods, which trainees were expected to use in their classrooms. They included the following:

- Effective methods to enhance participants' understanding of their feelings and values through individual and group discussions.

- Behavioral methods to help participants develop skills and practice what they learn. An example is role-play.

- Cognitive methods to provide information, stimulate the gathering of information and ideas, and encourage the learning of concepts. Examples include brainstorming, presentations by guest speakers, and use of charts, posters, books, and videos.

- Introspective methods to help participants see the relevance for their own lives of what they learn. Examples including writing a journal on the content and process of training/learning.

- Anonymous questions to provide participants the opportunity to ask questions they might be embarrassed to ask aloud. The number of anonymous questions declined during the course of the training, as trainees became more comfortable about the issues discussed and began to ask questions in class.

- Games to increase the comfort level of participants with sexual activities and body parts. In the Word Game, names of body parts are written on piece of a cardboard and participants are asked to read them aloud.

Training of master trainers

Twenty master trainers were selected from the pool of trained teachers, based on the following criteria:

- Excellent performance during the teaching practicum

- Excellent performance on the posttraining test of knowledge and attitudes

- Leadership qualities and keen interest in the subject demonstrated during training.

The program aimed to have a balance of male and female master trainers, although more women than men teach FLHE.

Training of master trainers lasted two days. It focused on increasing knowledge of FLHE concepts, the ability to make appropriate use of facilitation skills and aids, and comfort levels in discussing FLHE topics.

Training of master trainers took place in 2003 and 2005 (refresher training). During the refresher training, each master trainer facilitated a session and received feedback from other master trainers.

In 2005 these trainers provided FLHE training to more than 1,000 carrier subject teachers. Since then another 36 master trainers have been trained.

Curricular Approach, Time Allocation, and Student Assessment

FLHE is integrated into the regular curriculum of junior-secondary schools within two main carrier subjects, integrated science and social studies. FLHE is taught to all students in grades JS1–JS3. Up to three periods of 35–40 minutes a week are spent on FHLE. Content covers five main themes: human development, personal skills, HIV infection, relationships, and society and culture. Specific topics include behavior that puts people at risk of getting STIs or HIV; sexual abuse (forms, effects, prevention, sources of help); and stigmatization and discrimination of people living with or affected by HIV/AIDS.

Depending on the learning objective, one of the following activities is selected:

- Group discussions and activities

- Role-plays

- Lectures

- Brainstorming

- Discussion of gender issues

- Drama, sketches or plays

- Songs

- Games

- Skill-building activities

A class aimed at influencing behavior change, for instance, would use group discussions and role-play. A session aimed at increasing knowledge would use brainstorming or a lecture.

On the activities of the program

Those found to be more effective:

- Group discussions, because young people hear the views expressed by their peers and learn from each other.
- Skill-building activities such as role-play, because it helps young people apply the information/skills learned.

And those found to be less effective:

- Generally lectures have not been very effective because young people don't like being "preached at"
- Videos cannot be used due to lack of necessary equipment in schools.

Program Manager and Implementers

Assessment of Learners

Assessment of students' knowledge, skills, and attitudes is an integral part of the FLHE program. During or after each lesson, progress and understanding are measured through question-and-answer sessions and assessment of student participation in role-play and group discussions. The curriculum provides an evaluation guide for each topic, specifying the knowledge students should have mastered. The LSMoE Scheme of Work states that formal testing should be carried out at the end of each term.

Monitoring and Evaluation of Instruction

A monitoring team made up of local education district inspectors and PP TESCOM staff was set up to ensure effective monitoring of teaching. Fifty-five local education district inspectors and PP TESCOM staff took part in training and learned how to use an assessment form to measure teacher performance. Staff were trained in data entry and analysis.

Management

The program was initially housed in the Curriculum Department of LSMoE, whose role was to recommend ways of integrating the subject into the existing curriculum and developing an integrated scheme of work for implementing the program. As time went on, it was considered strategic and practical to place the program under the overall guidance of the Office of the Honourable Commissioner of Education, under the direct supervision of the Directorate of Private Education and Special Programmes.

Once the Curriculum Department had completed its work, PP TESCOM selected the teachers to be trained; AHI facilitated the actual training. PP TESCOM was also responsible for communicating with teachers and monitoring their participation and performance.

Partnership

The Lagos State Ministry of Education is responsible for developing and implementing education policies in the state. It carries out its work through a number of organs, including the Office of the Honourable Commissioner; the Office of the Permanent Secretary; and the departments of basic education services, higher education, science and technology, private education and special programs, curriculum services, inspectorate, finance and administration, and accounts, as well as the policy implementation, public relations, and internal audit units. AHI provides technical and financial assistance and enables implementation of activities (through, for example, the organization of training workshops).

Disseminating Information and Providing Technical Support for Scaling Up the Program

Program staff coordinated the dissemination of information on FLHE with the aim of introducing it in other states in Nigeria. Efforts included (a) training United Nations Family Planning Association (UNFPA) master trainers, who were subsequently expected to train others in states where UNFPA is active and (b) sponsoring learning visits for education ministry officials from the states of Plateau, Enugu, Anambra, Abia, and Rivers.

National dissemination was conducted in January 2006 during a dinner event at the National Stakeholders Conference on Strengthening FLHE Implementation in Nigeria. The goal was to advocate for scaling up FLHE implementation in other states, using the Lagos State success story as a model. The event was attended by 200 people, including a representative of the minister of state; state directors of education; state heads of inspectorate departments; staff of the Lagos State AIDS Control Agency; HIV/AIDS desk officers from all 36 states and the Federal Capital Territory; staff of the federal Ministry of Education HIV/AIDS Unit; representatives of CSOs and initiatives such as Nigeria's Community Participation for Action in the Social Sector Project and the Global HIV/AIDS Initiative in Nigeria; resource people and agencies such as UNFPA, the British Council, UNICEF, and UNAIDS; and other agencies that support such initiatives. Key officials from the ministries of education of all 36 states and the Federal Capital Territory received copies of documents on baseline measures, evaluation, impact, and lessons learned.

The program was also promoted at the following events:

- The 2005 International Conference on HIV/AIDS and Sexually Transmitted Infections in Africa

- International training programs organized by the Africa Regional Sexuality Resource Centre, an initiative covering four of the most populous countries in Africa (Egypt, Kenya, Nigeria, and South Africa)

- The World Congress on Sexology, held in Montreal in 2005.

Evaluation

To document the need for FLHE education and to measure the effectiveness of the program, a needs assessment and baseline survey of student knowledge, attitudes, and reported sexual behavior was conducted among 2,466 students between the ages of 10 and 19. The assessment was carried out in 2002 by Philliber Research Associates, a New York consulting firm, in collaboration with LSMoE, AHI, and the International Women's Health Coalition.

Methodology and Key Findings of Baseline Study

Knowledge and attitude questions were developed to match the content and message of each module of the curriculum. Where possible, questions were included that had already been tested with students the same age. The questions were reviewed for cultural appropriateness and readability. In addition, the questionnaires were pilot tested among a group of Nigerians 11–13.

The questionnaire examined the following issues:

- Age at first intercourse (if sexually active)

- Number of partners

- Frequency of sexual intercourse

- Pregnancies

- Births

- Consistency and efficacy of contraception use

- Knowledge and attitude about HIV/AIDS.

LSMoE administered the survey to students. The students came from 23 schools from all five Lagos school districts. Schools were chosen randomly.

The study confirmed that education on sexuality and HIV/AIDS was urgently needed. The results showed that students lacked basic knowledge about their bodies and how to protect themselves from unwanted pregnancy and HIV and that most were curious about or interested in trying sex. Like their peers around the world, many students reported experiencing peer pressure to have sex.

The study confirmed that boys and girls behave differently and experience pressure differently. For example, only 60 percent of boys reported they would stop trying to have sex with a girl if she asked him to stop. Most students felt abstinence from sex was not a viable option. Furthermore, students who were sexually active did not use protection against pregnancy or STIs.

Key Findings of Curriculum Evaluation

An evaluation of the impact of the FLHE program on students was conducted in July 2005, two years after the program was introduced. Information was gathered through surveys and focus group discussions. The results indicated that students increased their knowledge of and attitudes about sexual health. It also indicated improvement in communication skills between boys and girls.

As a result of the program, students:

- demonstrated increases in knowledge about STIs and HIV/AIDS,

- understood the vocabulary of sexuality and health,

- understood the meaning and desirability of abstinence,

- increased their knowledge of personal hygiene, and

- showed increased awareness of the risk of early pregnancy.

Learners' attitudes also improved. The FLHE curriculum had a positive effect on students' knowledge of the rights of girls to refrain from sexual activity. Girls gained confidence in their right to be able to refuse sexual advances and reported being less easily intimidated. A majority of boys agreed that it is wrong to force a girl to have sexual relations. They also agreed that boys should refrain from sexual activity because they are too young, want to stay healthy, and do not want to anger or disappoint their families.

Students also increasingly reported wanting to delay having sex. As their knowledge grew, they perceived fewer reasons to have sex and more reasons not to. Students and teachers attributed this change largely to the strong abstinence message conveyed in classrooms.

Key Findings of Teacher Evaluation

In June 2004, 45 teachers from 15 schools were surveyed. Some of the teachers had been trained to use the FLHE curriculum, others had not. The majority of teachers had at least 10 years' teaching experience. The objective was to assess teachers' reactions to and implementation of the FLHE curriculum and their comfort level in teaching it. In July 2005 focus group discussions with teachers and students were conducted to gain in-depth insight into survey responses.

The evaluation revealed several important findings:

- Some science teachers were offering topics that appear in the scheme of work for social studies, and some social studies teachers were teaching topics that appear in the scheme of work for integrated science.

- Skill-building activities were rarely included in lessons.

- Teachers were generally positive about FLHE.

- Teacher believed their students were less comfortable with discussing human sexuality than they themselves were.

Cost-Effectiveness

AHI provided $1.028 million, of which $825,000 was spent between 2003 and 2005. Based on this figure, the average cost per student was $2.58 over the three years of operations.

Lessons Learned

Several lessons emerged from the FLHE program.

Dealing with Opposition to the Program

A small organization has waged a campaign to keep the FLHE curriculum from being taught. In addition to using the media to decry the program, it sought to enlist political and other support to restrain both the federal government and the government of Lagos State from implementing FLHE in schools.

In recognition of the cultural sensitivity to sex education and to encourage public acceptance of the program, the program changed its name from the

"National Comprehensive Sexuality Education Curriculum Implementation Program" to the "National Family Life HIV/AIDS Education Curriculum Implementation Program." Teaching-learning contents were also adapted, leading to the removal from the curriculum of controversial topics such as the use of condoms.

Unfortunately, these changes did not assuage opposition to the program, which continues to provide misinformation to the mass media. To deal with this challenge, program officials try to explain the FLHE program and its value for young people at every possible opportunity.

Working around the Small Size of Classrooms

The large number of students and small size of most classrooms limits the ability to carry out interactive skill-building activities, which form the basis of effective teaching-learning about HIV/AIDS. A possible solution suggested by the program manager is to encourage teachers to conduct activities outside, on school premises.

Dealing with Limited Resources

The limited budget and general lack of resources leads to a range of challenges. To be fully effective, the program needs more trained teachers, better facilities, and more teaching-learning materials, particularly for students. The limited budget also affects the program's capacity to improve its public relations' component.

The shortage of trained teachers is being addressed in the ongoing FHLE teacher training program. Education on FHLE is also being integrated into tertiary teacher education at the preservice level.

Ensuring Uniform Mode of Delivery and Motivating Teachers

Teaching and comfort levels of teachers vary across schools. Most adhere to the lesson plan laid out in the scheme of work. On the whole, integrated science teachers are more comfortable teaching science-based aspects of sexuality, while social studies teachers focus more on the moral and social dimensions.

The program tries to motivate teachers through nonmonetary incentives, such as awarding training certificates, involving teachers in implementation processes, publicly acknowledging teachers' contributions, recognizing outstanding performances during award ceremonies, distributing resource materials to outstanding teachers, providing transportation allowances for meetings, and allowing some teachers to share their experiences in other states.

Conclusion

The FLHE program has enabled thousands of students across Lagos State to learn about HIV/AIDS. While cultural and political factors have meant that programmers have been unable to include every aspect of teaching that was initially intended, sensible compromise has enabled teaching of many program objectives to occur at a mass scale.

Several factors contributed to the success of the FLHE program:

- LSMoE recognized the need to involve partners to meet the demands imposed by the scale of the HIV epidemic in Nigeria.

- The program was developed based on a series of needs assessments.

- The program recognized and actively addressed the cultural diversity within Nigeria by including a wide range of stakeholders in the development of the program and teaching materials.

- Curriculum experts were involved in developing the FLHE curriculum.

Annex 10.1

ELPE Attainment of Impact Benchmarks

BENCHMARK	ATTAINMENT/COMMENTS
1. Identifies and focuses on specific sexual health goals	✓ Program aims to meet the sexual and reproductive health needs of young people. Specific objectives include reducing teenage pregnancy and STI and HIV transmission.
2. Focuses narrowly on specific behaviors that lead to sexual health goals	✓ Program focuses on, among other issues, increasing age of first intercourse and marriage and reducing teenage pregnancy and STI/HIV infection.
3. Identifies and focuses on sexual psychosocial risk and protective factors that are highly related to each of these behaviors	Partial. Program contents were shaped partly by findings of a learning needs assessment. Program aims to respond to needs by helping students acquire skills needed to make healthy decisions about their sexual health and behavior. Although young people indicated that they do not consider abstinence a viable option, the program promotes total abstinence.
4. Implements multiple activities to change each of the selected risk and protective factors	✓ Program uses variety of methods aimed at attaining cognitive, affective, and behavioral learning goals.
5. Actively involves youth by creating a safe social environment	✓ Learners are actively involved in classroom sessions, monitoring, and pretesting of teaching aids.

(*Continues on the following page*)

BENCHMARK	ATTAINMENT/COMMENTS
6. Employs a variety of teaching methods designed to involve participants and have them personalize the information	✓ Teaching methods employed—in particular the affective and behavioral methods—are designed to support student involvement and help students explore their own values related to sexual and reproductive health.
7. Conveys clear message about sexual activity and condom or contraceptive use and continually reinforces that message	Partial. Program focuses on abstinence. Safer sex is not included in the curriculum.
8. Includes effective curricula and activities appropriate to the age, sexual experience, and culture of participating students	Partial. Curriculum is structured by grade. Curriculum underwent changes because of cultural sensitivity over certain topics. As a result, it may be reflect the values of religious groups and other adults rather than those of young people.
9. Increases knowledge by providing basic, accurate information about the risks of teen sexual activity and methods of avoiding intercourse or using protection against pregnancy and STIs	Partial. Information on transmission and prevention of infection is provided. Condoms are not discussed as means of preventing pregnancy or disease.
10. Uses some of the same strategies to change perceptions of peer values, to recognize peer pressure to have sex, and to address that pressure	✓ Program addresses peer pressure and how to deal with it. In the lesson on negotiation skills and assertiveness, students learn skills for dealing with peer pressure.
11. Identifies specific situations that might lead to sex, unwanted sex, or unprotected sex and identifies methods of avoiding those situations or getting out of them	Partial. Curriculum deals with sexual abuse and what to do in case of abuse. It does not address negotiating safe sex.
12. Provides modeling of and practice with communication, negotiation, and refusal skills to improve both skills and self-efficacy in using those skills	✓ Program pays great deal of attention to self-esteem, goal setting, communication, and negotiation skills.

Source: Authors.

Annex 10.2

Contact Information

The Honourable Commissioner
Lagos State Ministry of Education
Mrs. J. O. Oshun, Permanent Secretary
P.M.B. 21043, Ikeja, Lagos, Nigeria
Tel: 01-4964787

Action Health Incorporated
Mrs. Nike O. Esiet, Executive Director
P.O. Box 803 Yaba, Lagos, Nigeria
Tel: 01-7743745, 01-7910402
Fax: 234-1-3425496
E-mail: info@actionhealthinc.org
Web site: www.actionhealthinc.org

Notes

1. Established in 1989, AHI is dedicated to improving the health of Nigerian adolescents. It has worked with young people; communities; and opinion leaders, including parents, local and national government staff, and policy makers, creating awareness and implementing programs to bring about change in the health status of adolescents in Nigeria.

2. In groups in which teachers displayed (particular) discomfort with the material, additional effort was made to help give them confidence in addressing the issues raised.

Appendix

Table A.1: Overview of Programs in the Dominican Republic, Eritrea, The Gambia, Ghana, and Israel

FEATURE	DOMINICAN REPUBLIC: PROGRAMA DE EDUCACION AFECTIVO SEXUAL (PEAS)	ERITREA: RAPID RESULTS INITIATIVE (RRI)	THE GAMBIA: INTEGRATED SECTORWIDE HIV/AIDS PREVENTIVE EDUCATION	GHANA: SCHOOL HEALTH EDUCATION PROGRAM (SHEP)	ISRAEL: JERUSALEM AIDS PROJECT (JAIP)
Goals, target groups, and policy framework					
Goal	Improve knowledge and practices of students and teachers to enable them to combat HIV/AIDS	Reduce transmission and impact of HIV among youth	Enable education sector to play a role in stemming tide of pandemic	Facilitate creation of well-informed and healthy school population	Reduce spread of HIV among young people, increase acceptance of people living with HIV/AIDS, reduce discrimination
Main focus	Provision of sex education with strong component on sexually transmitted infections and HIV/AIDS	Use of management tool to deliver school-based HIV/AIDS education	Effective coordination of education sector HIV/AIDS prevention activities	Setting of national standards for HIV/AIDS and school-based health education; coordination of efforts of NGOs	Provision of extracurricular HIV/AIDS education by volunteers
Main target group	Public secondary-school students	Junior- and secondary-school students in government schools	4- to 19-year-olds (HIV/AIDS education begins at age 7)	Students in preprimary, primary, and secondary schools	13- to 21-year-olds in primary and secondary schools and informal educational settings
Coverage	Students in 825 secondary schools	More than 40,000 students in 48 schools	All basic, upper-basic, and senior-secondary schools	All government schools have opportunity to participate	About 60 schools a year, reaching 30,000 students in 2004
Policy framework	Education activities referred to in national strategic plan and other legislation	In line with education sector policy on HIV/AIDS	In line with national education policy	Education activities are referred to in national HIV/AIDS policy	Not set in policy framework
Program implementation					
Coordinator	Department of Counseling and Psychology in State Secretariat of Education	Ministry of Education	HIV/AIDS unit within the Department of State for Education	School Health Education Program (unit of Ghana Education Service)	JAIP
Curricular approach	Infusion into regular curriculum; sex education lessons	Extracurricular	Integration of HIV/AIDS teaching into main carrier subject (Population and Family Life Education [POP/FLE])	Infusion into regular curriculum; co- and extracurricular activities	Extracurricular

Time allocation	One 30- to 50-minute lesson a week throughout the year	90–120 minutes a week	Program taught 45–60 minutes a week. One module of POP/FLE addresses HIV	Peer education takes place weekly during four-week period	Four academic hours spread over a minimum of two days
Average length of participation in program	Four years	At least 100 days	12 years	10 years	Most students are exposed to program five times: once in primary school, two or three times in secondary school, and once during army service
Role of NGOs/education sector partners	World Bank's Global AIDS Monitoring and Evaluation Team provides technical support for evaluation survey	Robert H. Schaffer & Associates provides technical support, UNICEF trains lead trainers in life skills	Nova Scotia–Gambia Association implements peer education program activities, United Nations Population Fund developed POP/FLE	Donors provide support; NGOs, community-based organizations, and faith-based organizations involved in program implementation	JAIP manages project
Collaboration with other sectors	Intersectoral partners support implementation	Intersectoral partners support implementation	Activities implemented primarily by education sector	Intersectoral partners support implementation	JAIP contracted by Ministry of Health to run AIDS hotline
Adaptation of program to other contexts	None	None	Program operates in coordination with other countries in region	None	Program adapted for use in 28 countries
Community involvement	Parents and other community members involved	Parents and other community members involved	Parents and other community members involved	Parents and other community members involved	Parents, communities, and religious organizations involved
Access to health services	Not included in program	Not included in program	Not included in program	Not included in program	Not included in program
Training and materials					
Teacher training and support					
Preservice training	Not included in program	Not included in program	Covers HIV/AIDS within POP/FLE curriculum; peer health educators active at Gambia Teacher Training College	Being developed	Not included in program

(Continues on the following page)

Table A.1: Overview of Programs in the Dominican Republic, Eritrea, The Gambia, Ghana, and Israel (continued)

FEATURE	DOMINICAN REPUBLIC: PROGRAMA DE EDUCACION AFECTIVO SEXUAL (PEAS)	ERITREA: RAPID RESULTS INITIATIVE (RRI)	THE GAMBIA: INTEGRATED SECTORWIDE HIV/AIDS PREVENTIVE EDUCATION	GHANA: SCHOOL HEALTH EDUCATION PROGRAM (SHEP)	ISRAEL: JERUSALEM AIDS PROJECT (JAIP)
In-service training	National, regional, and provincial sensitization activities; training of secondary-school teachers; some refresher training	After initial sensitization, teachers receive weekly training from program coaches; teachers provide weekly training of peer educators	Periodic training of trainers, teachers, guidance and counseling teachers, peer health educators, and Department of State for Education staff	Periodic training of SHEP national office staff, district coordinators, teachers, peer educators, and community members	Periodic training of teachers, school nurses, and NGO staff
Teaching-learning methods and activities	Wide range of participatory methodologies	Wide range of participatory methodologies	Program focuses on building knowledge about HIV; complementary activities concentrate on building skills and attitudes using various participatory methods	Wide range of participatory methodologies	Wide range of participatory methodologies
Peer education	Not part of program	Peer educators main agents of educational delivery to students	Part of program	Part of program	Provided by university students
Program materials	Manuals for teacher training; manuals for use by teachers, students, parents, and communities; supplementary materials	Manuals for trainers, teachers, and peer educators; activity sheets for peer educators; brochures and magazines to promote program	Teacher training manuals, teacher guides, assessment materials, guidance and counseling manual, student manual, student books, peer health educator manual	Implementation guidelines, HIV/AIDS–related curricula, teacher manuals, peer educator manuals, PTA manual, posters, leaflets, booklets	Educational kits for primary- and secondary-school students, including teacher guide, cartoons, flip charts, booklets, posters, stickers, condoms, and pre- and postintervention questionnaires; supplementary materials

Assessment

Assessment of needs				
Not conducted	Baseline and follow-up evaluation of knowledge, attitudes, and practices conducted for each phase of program	Not conducted	Not conducted	Conducted by experts in public health, education, and other fields
Assessment of teaching and learning progress				
Informal evaluations of student progress conducted	Informal evaluations of student progress conducted	Formal assessment conducted through examinations every term; informal assessment conducted for each program level	Informal evaluations of student progress conducted	Knowledge, attitudes, and practices questionnaire used at beginning and end of program
Monitoring and evaluation of implementation and outcomes				
Survey of knowledge of, attitudes toward, and practices related to STIs, HIV/AIDS, and sex education conducted in 2004 among students and secondary-school teachers to evaluate the program	Baseline and follow-up evaluations guide each phase of program	Monitoring of curricular activities by Department of State for Education's supervision and inspection unit; coordinators and trainers from Nova Scotia–Gambia Association monitor progress of delivery of program by peer health educators	Standards for HIV education activities defined leading to certification and awards, depending on progress of schools	Pre- and postintervention questionnaires administered to parents and students who participate in classes
Opinion of learners				
Not systematically solicited	Questionnaires administered to teachers and learners about program process	Not systematically solicited	Not systematically solicited	Informal assessment of student needs conducted during sessions
Program content				
Sexual and reproductive health				
Included	Included to limited degree	Included	Included	Included to limited degree
STIs and HIV/AIDS				
Included	Included	Included	Included	Included
Life skills				
Included	Included	Included	Included	Included

(Continues on the following page)

Table A.1: Overview of Programs in the Dominican Republic, Eritrea, The Gambia, Ghana, and Israel (continued)

FEATURE	DOMINICAN REPUBLIC: PROGRAMA DE EDUCACION AFECTIVO SEXUAL (PEAS)	ERITREA: RAPID RESULTS INITIATIVE (RRI)	THE GAMBIA: INTEGRATED SECTORWIDE HIV/AIDS PREVENTIVE EDUCATION	GHANA: SCHOOL HEALTH EDUCATION PROGRAM (SHEP)	ISRAEL: JERUSALEM AIDS PROJECT (JAIP)
Values/attitudes	Included	Included	Included	Included	Included
Social and cultural context of HIV/AIDS	Included	Included	Included	Included	Included
Gender relations	Included	Included	Included	Not specified	Not specified
Stigmatization and discrimination	Included	Included	Not specified	Not specified	Included
Funding and costs					
Funding source	World Bank	World Bank	Canadian International Development Agency provided funding for peer education through Nova Scotia–Gambia Association; UNICEF and United Nations Population Fund funded development of program materials	Donors (UNICEF, WHO, DANIDA, DfID, JICA, and USAID)	Ministry of Education and Ministry of Health
Annual cost	Not available	Teachers: $86 per phase Students: $19 per phase	Wide range of activities prevents simple cost breakdown	Not available	$1.72 per student in 2004
Main challenges					
Educator recruitment and turnover	Not an issue	Not an issue	Ongoing challenge	Not an issue	Recruitment of volunteers ongoing challenge
Program resources	Materials and training need improvement	Not an issue	Not an issue	Donor support limited to certain areas and schools	Not an issue
Integration of HIV/AIDS education into curriculum	Not an issue	Not an issue	Not an issue	Not an issue	Not an issue

Uniformity of implementation	Not an issue	Not an issue	Some schools sustain peer education well, others struggle	Program actively seeks to ensure consistency of implementation by many stakeholders	Not an issue
Teaching load	Too few trained teachers to cover all schools	Not an issue	Not an issue	Not an issue	Not an issue
Clarity of messages	Misperceptions and myths remain deeply entrenched	Not an issue	Some teachers have misconceptions about HIV	Not an issue	Not an issue
Commitment of various actors	Not an issue	Not an issue	Not an issue	Not an issue	Not an issue
Resistance to program	Not an issue	Not an issue	By religious authorities	Keeping motivation high when HIV prevalence is low is challenging	By religious authorities
Monitoring and evaluation	Requires strengthening	Long-term impact uncertain	Not an issue	Lack of funds for travel limits monitoring activities	Not an issue
Availability of relevant HIV/AIDS–related data	Not an issue	Not an issue	Not an issue	Not an issue	Not an issue
Sustainability	Improved program management needed	Not an issue	Not an issue	Not an issue	Recruitment of volunteers poses a problem
Adaptation to other contexts/countries	Not an issue	Not an issue	Not an issue	Not an issue	Program readily adapted to wide range of contexts in 28 countries
Other	Greater community involvement needed	Strong political leadership needed to maintain momentum	Peer educators may be of only limited efficacy	Not specified	Complacency about HIV/AIDS; keeping program up to date

Table A.2: Overview of Programs in Kenya, Namibia, and Nigeria

Goals, target groups, and policy framework

	KENYA: PRIMARY SCHOOL ACTION FOR BETTER HEALTH (PSABH)	KENYA: PRIMARY SCHOOL AIDS PREVENTION PROGRAM (PSAPP)	NAMIBIA: WINDOW OF HOPE (WOH)	NIGERIA: EXPANDED LIFE PLANNING EDUCATION (ELPE), OYO STATE	NIGERIA: FAMILY LIFE HIV/AIDS EDUCATION, (FLHE), LAGOS STATE
Goal	Reduce risk of HIV infection among upper-primary-school students by providing accurate information and enabling behavior change	Reduce spread of HIV among young people in Kenya and beyond	Develop resilience and self-esteem among upper-primary-school children to enable them to face challenges of society, including HIV/AIDS	Improve sexual and reproductive health of in-school youth in Oyo State and serve as model for national replication	Improve sexual and reproductive health status of young people in Lagos State
Main focus	Provision of HIV education	Evaluation of interventions aimed at preventing HIV and teenage pregnancy	Provision of HIV/AIDS education through extracurricular activities	Integration and teaching of ELPE in Oyo State secondary-school curriculum	Provision of education within school curriculum
Main target group	12- to 16-year-olds in upper-primary school	12- to 16-year-olds in grades 5–8	9- to 14-year-olds in primary school	9- to 20-year-olds in school	9- to 13-year-olds in first three years of junior secondary school
Coverage	5,000 out of 19,000 primary schools	328 primary schools in two districts	17,930 students in 37 percent of country's public primary schools	About 40 percent of secondary schools in Oyo State (more than 425,000 students)	All public junior-secondary schools in Lagos State (about 320,000 students)
Policy framework	Not specified	Not specified	National HIV/AIDS policy for education sector	Not specified	National Council on Education resolution on education sector response to HIV/AIDS

Program implementation

Coordination	Centre for British Teachers in cooperation with Ministry of Education, Science and Technology and Ministry of Health	Ministry of Education, Science and Technology; National AIDS Control Council; International Child Support	HIV/AIDS Management Unit within Ministry of Basic Education, Sports and Culture	Three governmental organs (Ministry of Education, Science and Technology; Ministry of Health; and Teaching Service Commission) and one NGO (Association for Reproductive and Family Health)	Lagos State Ministry of Education

Curricular approach	Main carrier subject (physical education) and infusion into other subjects; co- and extracurricular activities	Sugar daddy talk, essay writing, debating	Extracurricular clubs	Taught as stand-alone subject as part of secondary-school curriculum	Integrated into two main carrier subjects (integrated science and social studies)
Time allocation	One hour a week in physical education	40–60 minutes a week	One lesson period a week	One hour a week during all four years of secondary schooling	One to three 35- to 40-minute periods a week
Average length of participation in program (years)	Four	Varies	Four	Four	Three
Role of NGOs/education sector partners	Ministry of Education, Science and Technology coordinated policy environment; Kenya Institute of Education developed materials	International Child Support coordinated implementation; UNICEF provided materials; Poverty Action Lab (MIT) coordinated evaluation	UNICEF provided technical support	Association for Reproductive and Family Health has overall responsibility for project; executive director is project coordinator and chief accounting officer	Action Health Incorporated provided technical and financial support; Philliber Research Associates provided technical support for needs assessment
Collaboration with other sectors	Ministry of Health supports training	Activities implemented primarily by education sector	Activities implemented primarily by education sector	Intersectoral cooperation important feature of program	Activities implemented primarily by education sector
Adaptation of program to other contexts	None	None	None	Replicated in Kebbi, Bauchi, Gombe, Yobe, and Borne states	None
Community involvement	Parents and other community members involved	Not included in program	Parents and other community members involved	Parents and other community members involved	Wide range of stakeholders contributed to review of curriculum
Access to health services	Not included in program	Not included in program	Not included in program	Youth-friendly health centers established in primary health care centers	Not included in program
Training and materials					
Teacher training and support					
Preservice training	In development	Not included in program	Not included in program	Not included in program	In development

(Continues on the following page)

229

Table A.2: Overview of Programs in Kenya, Namibia, and Nigeria (continued)

	KENYA: PRIMARY SCHOOL ACTION FOR BETTER HEALTH (PSABH)	KENYA: PRIMARY SCHOOL AIDS PREVENTION PROGRAM (PSAPP)	NAMIBIA: WINDOW OF HOPE (WOH)	NIGERIA: EXPANDED LIFE PLANNING EDUCATION (ELPE), OYO STATE	NIGERIA: FAMILY LIFE HIV/AIDS EDUCATION, (FLHE), LAGOS STATE
In-service training	Sensitization of key stakeholders; strengthened cascade training for teachers, peer educators, and community representatives	Teacher training	Teacher training, followed by refresher training for trainers and teachers; regional resource centers provide access to information on HIV/AIDS; cluster meetings allow exchange of experiences	Training of trainers, supervisors, health care providers; school-level training includes training of teachers and peer educators; teacher refresher course periodically provided	Sensitization of key stakeholders; training of master trainers and carrier subject teachers; refresher training
Teaching-learning methods and activities	Wide range of participatory methodologies	Range of participatory methodologies	Wide range of participatory methodologies	Wide range of participatory methodologies	Wide range of participatory methodologies
Peer education	Part of program	Not part of program	Not part of program	Part of program	Not part of program
Program materials	Teacher manuals, classroom materials, peer educator materials, school health club kit	UNICEF teaching materials	Not included in program	Training and support materials; materials for use by teachers; materials for use by students and other young people; information, education, and communication materials	National FLHE curriculum, teaching-learning materials, resource manuals
Assessment					
Assessment of needs	Conducted in 1999	Study of teachers conducted in 2002 guided design of program	National study conducted in 2003 by Ministry of Basic Education, Sports and Culture and the National Institute of Education Development	Study of student needs conducted in Oyo State in 1998 by Association for Reproductive and Family Health	Conducted in 2003
Assessment of teaching and learning progress	No formal assessment of progress conducted	Formal assessment through essay writing, informal assessment of sugar daddy activities	Not yet implemented	No formal assessment of progress conducted	Formal testing conducted at end of each term

Monitoring and evaluation of implementation and outcomes	Program includes rigorous schedule of evaluation activities	Stratified randomized evaluation of four different interventions used; cost-effectiveness research conducted	Monitoring system not yet operational	Life-planning education coordinator supervises daily; zonal and local education inspectors monitor monthly; Ministry of Education, Science and Technology project coordinating unit monitors bimonthly; program partners monitor quarterly; teachers and peer educators use management information system forms	Team composed of local inspectors and teaching service commission staff monitors implementation
Opinion of learners	Not systemically solicited	Not systemically solicited	Not systemically solicited	Not systemically solicited	Not systemically solicited
Program content					
Sexual and reproductive health	Included	Included	Included	Included	Included
STIs and HIV/AIDS	Included	Included	Included	Included	Included
Life skills	Included	Included	Included	Included	Included
Values/attitudes	Included	Not specified	Included	Included	Included
Social and cultural context of HIV/AIDS	Included	Included	Not specified	Included	Included
Gender relations	Included	Not specified	Included	Included	Included
Stigmatization and discrimination	Not included	Not specified	Included	Not specified	Not specified
Other	Guidance and counseling	Not specified	Development of sense of belonging among family, friends, and school	Improvement in parent/child education; building of poverty-reduction/income-generation skills	Not specified

(Continues on the following page)

Table A.2: Overview of Programs in Kenya, Namibia, and Nigeria (continued)

	KENYA: PRIMARY SCHOOL ACTION FOR BETTER HEALTH (PSABH)	KENYA: PRIMARY SCHOOL AIDS PREVENTION PROGRAM (PSAPP)	NAMIBIA: WINDOW OF HOPE (WOH)	NIGERIA: EXPANDED LIFE PLANNING EDUCATION (ELPE), OYO STATE	NIGERIA: FAMILY LIFE HIV/AIDS EDUCATION, (FLHE), LAGOS STATE
Funding and costs					
Funding source	DfID; Ministry of Education, Science and Technology; Ministry of Health	Partnership for Child Development, World Bank	UNICEF, Ministry of Basic Education, Sports and Culture	DfID supported development and implementation in Oyo State; Ford Foundation provided support for expansion to other states	Action Health Incorporated, World Bank
Annual cost per student	$3.18 ($5.79 where peer educators trained)	Teacher training: $2.00; debate and essay writing: $1.10; sugar daddy talk: $0.80; school uniforms: $12	$30.60	$1.80	$2.58
Main challenges					
Educator recruitment and turnover	Teacher and peer educator turnover high	Not an issue	Teacher turnover high	Teacher transfer a challenge	Not an issue
Program resources	Sufficient	Sufficient	Lack of trained teachers	Sufficient	Lack of trained teachers; training and materials need improvement
Integration of HIV/AIDS education into curriculum	Not an issue	Not an issue	Not an issue	Curriculum is overcrowded, implementation depends on school	Not an issue
Uniformity of implementation	Need to ensure that messages received in school are consistent with those received out of school is challenge	Not an issue	Not an issue	Not an issue	Teachers have different levels of comfort in teaching curriculum
Teaching load	Not an issue	Not an issue	Teachers overburdened by HIV initiatives	Teachers complain of being overstretched	Not an issue

Adaptation to different age and cultural groups	Not an issue	Not an issue	English, the language of all program materials, is not first language of many participating children	Not an issue	Not an issue
Clarity of messages	Not an issue	Not an issue	Not an issue	Not an issue	Not an issue
Commitment of various actors	Not an issue	Not an issue	Not an issue	Students did not take subject as seriously as other, examinable subjects	Not an issue
Resistance to program	Not an issue	Not an issue	Not an issue	Not an issue	Opposition from some religious groups
Monitoring and evaluation	Not an issue	Not an issue	Evaluation not yet implemented	Not an issue	Not an issue
Availability of relevant HIV/AIDS–related data	Not an issue	Not an issue	Overflow of HIV information makes it difficult for teachers to make informed choices	Not an issue	Not an issue
Sustainability	Program has minimized payments to teachers to maximize sustainability	Not an issue	Political changes and commitment may affect program's sustainability	Provision of ongoing funding uncertain	Not an issue
Other	Not specified	Not specified	Not specified	Differences between government and NGO cultures; public sector strikes in education and health	Small size of classrooms make use of interactive methodologies difficult

Index

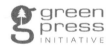